"This volume answers the question: how can psychoanalysts help our troubled world? Through the leadership of the IPA in the Humanitarian Field Committee, the reader is introduced to a global collection of creative, effective, psychoanalytic efforts to restore a sense of humanity, of physical, cultural, and psychic containment, to refugees and migrants. The task of truly hearing stories of exploitation, torture, and loss – of homeland, language, community, socioeconomic position, health, and safety – requires the ability to listen deeply while holding intense effect. Every person who wants to help fellow citizens of the world impacted by current crises of climate, social injustice, economic inequity, and political oppression will benefit from the psychological and systems insights offered by the psychoanalyst authors of *Trauma, Flight and Migration*."

Harriet Wolfe, *MD, president, International Psychoanalytical Association*

"Studying traumatizing world events from a psychoanalytic angle is a difficult task. However, such an investigation not only offers new treatment options for those who suffered but also informs authorities on how to deal with societal, political, and economic approaches to such an event. This book brings together psychoanalysts around the world who address the largest refugee problems we are presently facing. We learn what clinical psychoanalysis can offer in improving the care of traumatized newcomers, including children. Another objective is the sharing of psychoanalytically informed data with humanitarian organizations and the UN. The COVID-19 pandemic led to more preoccupation with physical borders between the nation states complicating illegal refugee issues. This book is most timely."

Vamık Volkan, *MD, emeritus professor of psychiatry, University of Virginia; emeritus president, International Dialogue Initiative; author of* Large-Group Psychology: Racism, Societal Divisions, Narcissistic Leaders and Who We Are Now

"This book demonstrates how psychoanalytic knowledge can contribute in important ways to understand and deal with the challenges posed by the unprecedented number of migrants and refugees seeking asylum today because of war, civil unrest, and economic turmoil in their homeland countries. In a unique way, and with impressive examples from psychoanalysts' worldwide work of engaging in societal issues, the book provides in-depth knowledge about relational problems, identity crises and unconscious conflicts resulting from severe trauma, violence, kidnaping, trafficking, and separation from families. Being a tribute to

IPA's increasing commitment to comprehend the political, social, and cultural context of mental health problems, this book, dealing with the deeply upsetting reality of flight, migration, and exile, is of interest for a wide audience."

Siri Erika Gullestad, *professor emeritus, University of Oslo; training analyst and past president of the Norwegian Psychoanalytic Society; chair of IPA Research Committee*

Trauma, Flight and Migration

This book brings together leading international psychoanalysts to discuss what psychoanalysis can offer to people who have experienced trauma, flight, and migration.

The four parts of the book cover several elements of this work, including psychoanalytic projects beyond the couch, and collaboration with the UN. Each chapter presents an example of the applications of psychoanalysis with a specific group or in a particular context, from working with refugees in China to understanding the experiences of women who have witnessed political violence in Peru. Psychoanalytic work within *Trauma, Flight and Migration* provides a compelling exploration of the international contributions made by psychoanalysis.

This innovative book will be essential reading for psychoanalysts and psychoanalytic psychotherapists looking to learn more about working with people who have experienced the impact of traumatic movement or migration.

Vivienne Elton, MBBS, DPM, FRANZCP, is a psychiatrist and psychoanalyst, past president and current training analyst of the Australian Psychoanalytical Society, and chair of the IPA in the Humanitarian Field Committee.

Marianne Leuzinger-Bohleber, MD, Dr. phil., is former professor for psychoanalysis at the University of Kassel and director of the Sigmund-Freud-Institut, Frankfurt a.M. She is currently senior professor at the University Medicine Mainz, training analyst of the German Psychoanalytical Association (DPV/IPA), vice chair of the Research Board of the IPA (2010–2021), and member and former chair of the IPA Subcommittee for Migration and Refugees.

Gertraud Schlesinger-Kipp, Dr. phil., is a psychologist, psychoanalyst, training analyst of the German Psychoanalytical Association (DPV, IPA), and chair of the IPA Subcommittee for Migration and Refugees.

Vivian B. Pender, MD, is clinical professor of psychiatry, Weill Cornell Medical College, and training psychoanalyst at Columbia University. She has chaired the UN Committee of the International Psychoanalytical Association since 2009.

IPA in the Community
Series editor: Harvey Schwartz

Recent titles in the series include:

Applying Psychoanalysis in Medical Care
Edited by Harvey Schwartz

Trauma, Flight and Migration
Psychoanalytic Perspectives
Edited by Vivienne Elton, Marianne Leuzinger-Bohleber,
Gertraud Schlesinger-Kipp, and Vivian B. Pender

Trauma, Flight and Migration
Psychoanalytic Perspectives

Edited by Vivienne Elton, Marianne Leuzinger-Bohleber, Gertraud Schlesinger-Kipp, and Vivian B. Pender

Routledge
Taylor & Francis Group

LONDON AND NEW YORK

Cover image: © Elly Brooks Photography. The image is from a folio on asylum-seeking refugees in Melbourne.

First published 2023
by Routledge
4 Park Square, Milton Park, Abingdon, Oxon OX14 4RN

and by Routledge
605 Third Avenue, New York, NY 10158

Routledge is an imprint of the Taylor & Francis Group, an informa business

British Library Cataloguing-in-Publication Data
A catalogue record for this book is available from the British Library

Library of Congress Cataloging-in-Publication Data
A catalog record for this book has been requested

ISBN: 978-1-032-03490-4 (hbk)
ISBN: 978-1-032-06652-3 (pbk)
ISBN: 978-1-003-20322-3 (ebk)

DOI: 10.4324/9781003203223

Typeset in Palatino
by Apex CoVantage, LLC

This book is dedicated to the migrants and refugees who fled war and trauma and have contributed much to their new countries and the many who live in hope. And to the late Robert Emde, himself a refugee, whose work to prevent the impact of early trauma was an inspiration to so many of us.

Contents

Editors and contributors

Vivienne Elton, MB, BS, DPM, FRANZCP, is a psychiatrist and psychoanalyst, past president and training analyst of the Australian Psychoanalytical Society, and chair of the IPA in the Humanitarian Field committee. She was a member of the Society Executive of the Australian Psychoanalytical Society for 12 years in various roles.

She has been chair of the IPA in the Humanitarian Field Committee since 2018, which includes the Migrants and Refugees and the IPA at the United Nations subcommittees.

Vivienne was visiting professor in the Huazhong University of Science and Technology, for the psychotherapy training programme in Wuhan, China, and is now a member of the IPA Sponsoring Committee for the China Study Group.

She supervises clinicians and teaches infant observation in China. From 2016 to 2019 she was President of the National Association of Practicing Psychiatrists in Australia working to improve and sustain available psychiatric, psychoanalytic, and psychotherapeutic treatments for the public. She is currently vice president of NAPP.

She has been involved in teaching in psychotherapeutic and psychoanalytic programmes for many years and has written curriculum with colleagues for the psychoanalytic training of APAS. She works in private practice in Victoria, Australia, as a psychoanalyst and has an interest in working with mothers and babies, migrants and refugees, survivors of war and genocide, and psychosomatics in psychoanalysis.

Professor Marianne Leuzinger-Bohleber, MD, Dr. phil., is director-in-charge of the Sigmund-Freud-Institut in Frankfurt a.M., Germany (2001–2016); professor emerita for psychoanalysis at the University of Kassel; and senior professor at the IDeA Excellency Center in Frankfurt a.M. and the University Medicine in Mainz. She is training analyst of the German Psychoanalytical Association (DPV) and the International Psychoanalytical Association (IPA). She was chair of the Committee for Research and Universities of the DPV (2001–2017); chair of the Research

Subcommittees for Clinical, Conceptual, Historical and Epistemological Research of the IPA (2001–2009); vice chair for Europe of the Research Board of the IPA (2010–2021). In 2018–2019 she was chair of the IPA Subcommittee for Migration and Refugees. She is still a member of this committee.

She received the Mary Sigourney Award 2016 and the Haskell Norman Prize for Excellence in Psychoanalysis 2017.

Her research fields are clinical and extra-clinical research in psychoanalysis, psychoanalytical developmental research, prevention studies, interdisciplinary dialogue between psychoanalysis and literature, educational sciences, and the neurosciences.

Vivian B. Pender, MD, DLFAPA, is a clinical professor of Psychiatry at the Weill Cornell Medical College and a training psychoanalyst at Columbia University. At the United Nations she represents the International Psychoanalytical Association and the American Psychiatric Association. A Distinguished Life Fellow, she serves as a trustee of the American Psychiatric Association. She served as the 148th President of the American Psychiatric Association. The theme of her 2021 presidency was social determinants of mental health, focusing on prevention of mental illness. She has honours and awards for her excellence teaching medical students, residents, and fellows. Until 2011 she chaired the NGO Committee on the Status of Women and is the immediate past chair of the NGO Committee on Mental Health, coalitions of non-governmental organisations in consultative status with the UN that include the APA and the IPA. As a UN consultant psychiatrist, she was instrumental in the establishment of UN Women. She is a volunteer asylum evaluator for Physicians for Human Rights. In 2015 she founded Healthcare against Trafficking Inc., a non-profit organisation dedicated to promoting education and advocacy in the health care sector. To this end she has presented grand rounds and symposia on the prevention of child abuse. She is a co-investigator on a Weill Cornell Department of Internal Medicine innovative grant to study "Experiences of Sex Trafficking Victims in Healthcare Settings." She produced four documentaries of conferences at the United Nations on mental health, human rights, human trafficking, and violence. She has published journal articles and book chapters on affect, pregnancy, sex trafficking, and leadership. In 2016 her edited book, *The Status of Women: Violence, Identity and Activism*, was published. She is currently working on two books titled *Healthcare against Sex Trafficking: Law, Medicine and Social Justice* and *Sexual Exploitation of Women and Children*. One of her current projects is to standardise a global psychiatry curriculum for graduate training. She is in private practice in New York City.

Gertraud Schlesinger-Kipp, Dr. phil., is a psychologist, psychoanalyst, and training analyst of the German Psychoanalytical Association (DPV,

IPA). She was president of the Alexander-Mitscherlich-Institute in Kassel and president of the DPV. In the IPA she was a member of the board. She founded the German part of the Committee on Women and Psychoanalysis (COWAP) in 2002 and was also overall chair of COWAP. Her main interest is the support of women through psychoanalysis, especially in emerging IPA areas (China, India, Georgia).

Now she is active in the committee "Migration and Refugees" of the IPA. She has authored numerous publications on "Female Development in Life Cycle," "Childhood in World War II," and psychotherapeutic approach with refugees.

Contributors

Paola Amendoeira is a psychologist with specialisation in mental health in childhood and adolescence by the Institute of Psychiatry of UFRJ (IPUB), an associate member of the Psychoanalysis Society of Brasilia, currently editor of the *Journal of the Psychoanalysis Society of Brasilia – Free Association*, and a member of the IPA's UN Committee.

Fabio Castriota, MD, lives and works in Rome as a private practitioner in psychiatry and psychoanalysis. He is a full member of the Italian Psychoanalytical Society (PSI) and is currently its vice president. He is also past president of the Roman Psychoanalytical Centre (CPdR) and lecturer at the SPI Training Institute and other Societies of Psychotherapy.

His main areas of interest are the study of dreams and the following relations: mind/body, psychoanalysis/neuroscience, psychoanalysis/art, and social situations.

His articles have been published in various reviews and books.

He is the focal point for the SPI group named PER (European Psychoanalysts for Refugees), which includes psychoanalysts dealing directly with refugee hospitality in Italy and with operators of this sector.

He presented the work "The Psychoanalysis and the Drama of Refugees" at the 50th International Psychoanalytic Association (IPA) Congress, held in Buenos Aires in 2017.

He was responsible for framework agreements between the Italian minister of health and SPI.

Anna L. Christopoulos, PhD, is a professor of clinical psychology and director of the graduate programme in clinical psychology in the National and Kapodistrian University of Athens, Greece. She is a full member of the Hellenic Psychoanalytic Association, the European Psychoanalytic Federation, and the International Psychoanalytic Association. She is a core member of the European Psychoanalytic Comparative Clinical Methods (CCM) moderators' group. She received her undergraduate degree in psychology from Brown University and her PhD in clinical psychology from New York University. She is also an associate board member of the *International Journal of Psychoanalysis*.

She is the author of the book *Introduction to Adult Psychopathology* (Topos Books) as well as numerous articles and book chapters.

Željko Čunović, is a psychiatrist and psychoanalyst in private practice; supervising and training analyst of the German Psychoanalytic Association/IPA; training analyst at the Anna-Freud-Institute, Frankfurt; member of Medico International Frankfurt since 1989; co-founder of *fatra* e.V. (Frankfurter Arbeitskreis Trauma und Exil) in 1993; professional director of the @Treatment Centre for Refugees and Victims of Torture (FATRA) until 2004; 2015 co-founder of the International Clinic at Frankfurt Psychoanalytic Institute (FPI); and currently director/chairman of the FPI.

Chrysi Giannoulaki, MD, PhD, is a psychiatrist and a training analyst of the Hellenic Psychoanalytic Association, and member of the European Psychoanalytic Federation and International Psychoanalytic Association. She is particularly interested in psychoses and narcissism. She is a full member of the Scientific Section *Psychiatry and Art* of the Hellenic Psychiatric Association and for many years has been involved in the organization of events that aim to enhance awareness of racism and xenophobia., such as film presentations followed by conferences, congresses etc. She is the author of the book *"Narcissism and Psychoanalysis-Heinz Kohut"* (in Greek) as well as numerous articles and book chapters.

Debra Gill, LCSW, is a training and supervising analyst at the Psychoanalytic Training Institute of the Contemporary Freudian Society, where she is on the permanent faculty. She teaches and supervises for the Metropolitan Institute for Training in Psychoanalytic Psychotherapy and through their continuing education programme offers seminars that reach the broader mental health community. She has presented papers on a number of panels for the IPA and ApsaA. Presently, she serves on both the IPA in the Humanitarian Field Committee and the Addictions Subcommittee.

Elizabeth Haworth is a psychoanalyst and member of the Peruvian Psychoanalytical Society with extensive experience in projects involving national and international cooperation. Her aim is to include a psychoanalytical understanding of the diversity and complexities of Peru's population through working on public policies (women, health, education) with the teams in charge of executing these policies. A psychologist from the Pontifical Catholic University of Peru, she has a diploma in gender and development from the International Development Research Center (IDRC) and Saint Mary's University, Halifax, Canada.

Nora Hettich, PhD, clinical psychologist and research assistant at the University of Kassel, has been one of the main coordinators of the STEP-BY-STEP programme. Dr Hettich wrote her PhD about psychosocial support for refugees at the University of Kassel and the Sigmund-Freud-Institut in Frankfurt, Germany. She is postdoc researcher at the Medical University Center Mainz and is currently in psychoanalytic training.

Sargam Jain, MD, is a psychiatrist and psychoanalyst with a specialisation in public mental health. Following completion of residency at Weill Cornell Medical Center, she did a fellowship in public psychiatry at the New York State Psychiatric Institute and completed psychoanalytic training at Columbia University and has been a Member of the Board of Trustees of the UN Voluntary Fund for Victims of Torture since September 2020. She is currently in private practice in Manhattan and on the medical school faculty at Weill Medical College of Cornell University, where she teaches community psychiatry to third-year residents.

Vladimir Jović, MD, PhD, is a psychiatrist, and psychoanalyst with private practice in Belgrade, training analyst of the Belgrade Psychoanalytical Society, and former president of the BPS (2014–2018). He works as a consultant of the Centre for Rehabilitation of Torture Victims (IAN) in Belgrade.

Gilbert Kliman, MD, is medical director of the Psychological Trauma Center, a division of the Children's Psychological Health Center; an adult, child, and adolescent psychiatrist who has focused on treatment and research concerning traumatised persons since before graduation from Harvard Medical School in 1953.

He is a Distinguished Life Fellow and Diplomate, American Psychiatric Association; Senior Life Fellow and Diplomate, Am. Academy Child & Adolescent Psychiatry; certified psychoanalyst for children, adolescents and adults – Am. Psychoanalytic Association; and medical director, Children's Psychological Health Center Inc.

Rosalba Maccarrone Erhardt is a psychologist and psychoanalyst and works in her own practice in Frankfurt/Main. She is a member of the DPV/IPA and since 2016 the head of the psychoanalytic outpatient clinic of the Frankfurt Psychoanalytic Institute (FPI), especially responsible for training in psychodynamic psychotherapy. She is a supervisor and coordinates the FPI-project "Help for Refugees" as a part of the "Psychosocial Network Rhein Main." From 2007 to 2020 she was a member of staff in the LAC- (Long-Term Therapy for Chronic Depression) Study.

David Morgan D. Clin. Psych, MSc, is a consultant psychotherapist and psychoanalyst; a fellow of the British Psychoanalytic Society; and training analyst and supervisor, BPA. He worked for many years in the National Health Service in the UK. He lectures internationally and nationally. He is chair of the Political Minds seminars at the Institute of

Psychoanalysis & Frontier Psychoanalyst on the UK radio. He is also the editor of "Violence Delinquency and Perversion" (Karnac) and has edited two new books in the Political Mind series. The first is out now: *The Role of the Unconscious in Social and Political Life* (Phoenix).

Maya Nadig, PhD, is a psychoanalyst and ethnologist from Zurich, was professor of ethnology at the University of Bremen at the "Institute for Ethnology and Cultural Studies" from 1991 to 2012. She focused on ethnopsychoanalysis, postcolonial cultural theories, migration, and transculturality. She has conducted much ethnopsychoanalytical research in Mexico, later in Switzerland, and more recently in China. Since 2010 she has made several visits to the matrilineal Mosuo culture in Southern China, where she sought to understand the forms of child-rearing and the nature of relationships. Her publications deal with psychodynamic processes in transcultural contexts, such as therapy with patients from other cultures. She is currently working as a psychoanalyst in practice.

Professor Joan Raphael-Leff (retired) is both an academic and clinician, Transcultural Psychologist and Psychoanalyst (Fellow of the British Psychoanalytical Society). Since qualification in 1976, she specialised in treating individuals and couples with Reproductive and early parenting issues. She is widely published 12 books and over 100 single authored peer-reviewed papers (translated into Chinese, Dutch, French, Flemish, Greek, Hebrew, Hungarian, Italian, Japanese, Polish, Portuguese, and Spanish).

In 1998 she founded COWAP, the IPA committee on Women & Psycho-analysis. Currently, She is Leader of Anna Freud Centre Academic Faculty for Psycho-analytic Research. Previously, she was head of University College London MSc in Psychoanalytic Developmental Psychology, and Professor of Psychoanalysis at the Centre for Psychoanalytic Studies at the University of Essex, UK and Stellenbosch University, South Africa.

As consultant to perinatal and women's projects she has supervised/lectured/taught in Argentina, Australia, Austria, Azores, Belgium, Canada, Canary Islands, Chile, China, Crete, Czech rep., Denmark, Egypt, England, Ethiopia, Finland, France, Germany, Greece, Guatemala, Holland, Hong Kong, India, Ireland, Israel, Italy, Japan, Latvia, Madeira, New Zealand, Madeira, Norway, Persia, Peru, Portugal, Russia, Scotland, South Africa, Spain, Sweden, Switzerland, Tobago, Trinidad, Turkey, USA, and Venezuela.

Laura Ravaioli, PhD, is a Psychologist Psychoanalyst of Società Psicoanalitica Italiana (SPI) and International Psychoanalytical Association. She has been a member of the I.P.A. Image Task Force and Public

Communication Committee. Since 2015 she has been a member of the I.P.A. Committee for the United Nations, and its co-chair since 2021.

Barbara Saegesser, PhD, is a training analyst with the Swiss Psychoanalytical Society and a member of the IPA. She has held several leadership positions in the Swiss Psychoanalytical Society and the Psychoanalytical Seminary of Basel. She is president of the commission treating ethical problems in the Swiss Society of Psychoanalysis. She has given papers at conferences and lectures in Switzerland, Germany, Ethiopia, and Djibouti. Since 2005 she has worked part time in ethnopsychoanalytical, psychoanalytical, psychotherapeutic, and training work in Eastern Islamic African cities and different Eastern African countries – that is, the poorest part of the dark continent: Alexandria (Egypt), Khartoum (Sudan), Addis Ababa and Hawassa (Ethiopia), Djibouti, Kampala (Uganda), and Zanzibar (Tanzania). Workplaces have included orphanages, with street boys, in baby shelters, hospital for the poorest, maternity (with third-degree genitally mutilated women), large orphanages and educational organisations, the central hospital of the island, and the psychiatric department. She has written publications and spoken at conferences on her Eastern African work.

Annabelle Starck is a psychologist in psychoanalytic training and research assistant at the Sigmund-Freud-Institut Frankfurt and also an employee at its outpatient department, as well as working at the Counselling and Therapy Center for Refugees at the Goethe-University Frankfurt. She has been engaged in the STEP-BY-STEP programme.

Johanna Mendoza Talledo is a psychoanalyst and current editor of the *Psychoanalysis* Journal of the Peruvian Society of Psychoanalysis (SPP) since 2018. She is a clinical psychologist, with a Master in Theoretical studies of Psychoanalysis and studies in the post-Doctoral program of Philosophy at the Pontifical Catholic University of Peru (PUCP). She was Scientific Secretary of the Peruvian Association of Psychoanalytic Psychotherapy of Children and Adolescents (APPPNA, 2009–2011), and Professor at the Peruvian Society of Psychoanalysis (SPP) Institute. She is the author of articles on female sexuality, gender and sexual diversity: Maternal genealogy: narcissistic identification in three generations of women. In *The Status of Women: Violence, Identity, and Activism* (2017). Editor Vivian Pender. Great Britain: Karnac. Co-editor of *Motherhood and its vicissitudes today* (2006). Lima: Sidea. Author of articles in the specialty of gender and psychoanalysis and in the work with Community and Culture.

Nicholas Tzavaras, MD, PhD, is a psychiatrist as well as a supervising and training analyst of the Hellenic Psychoanalytic Society in Athens, Greece. He was previous president of the Hellenic Psychoanalytic

Society as well as president of the Hellenic Psychiatric Association. He completed his medical studies at Universities of Bonn and Berlin. He specialised in neurology and psychiatry at the University of Giessen. He also completed his psychoanalytic training at the psychoanalytic Institute of Giessen and became a member of that institute. From 1987 until 2007 he was professor of psychiatry at the University of Thrace in Alexandroupolis, Greece. For the last 15 years he has been actively involved in cultural psychoanalysis and most recently with issues concerning immigrants and refugees in Greece and formed a Committee for Refugees in the Hellenic Psychoanalytic Society that offers therapy, supervision, and research.

Sverre Varvin, MD. Dr. Philos., is a member of the Norwegian Psychoanalytic Society. He is professor emeritus at the Oslo Metropolitan University. He has been working clinically and with research on traumatisation and the treatment of traumatised patients, especially in the refugee field. He has done process and outcome research on psychoanalytic therapy, research on traumatic dreams, and on psychoanalytic training. He has twice been president of the Norwegian Psychoanalytic Society, and he has had several positions in the IPA, among others as vice president and board member and chair of the IPA Working Group on Terror and Terrorism. He is presently chair of IPA China Committee.

He has published articles and books on traumatisation, refugees, terrorism, and on research on treatment process and outcome.

Book series introduction

I am pleased to welcome you to the IPA in the Community Book Series. These volumes will present the outreach work of the International Psychoanalytic Association as it integrates itself into many facets of our community life. We will learn how psychoanalysis, while born in the consulting room, also has application far beyond. Its core skills inform care provided to many individuals and in many venues from cancer units to refugee centres, from prenatal clinics to prisons. Through this book series we will get the opportunity to observe the deeply generous and skilful work of psychoanalysts who are making meaningful contact with individuals both on and off the couch.

Harvey Schwartz, MD
Series Editor

Foreword

The publication of this excellent book is as timely as it is necessary. It has been edited by four prestigious female psychoanalysts, who in addition to being well known in their profession have dedicated many years of their lives to working with migrants and refugees. At the beginning of the introduction, they inform us of the terrible figure of 82.4 million migrants and refugees who in 2021 have sought asylum in countries far from their cities of origin because of war, civil unrest, or economic turbulence.

The editors have gathered 18 testimonies of psychoanalysts who have managed to go beyond a discursive proposal by bringing the psychoanalytic method to concrete work with people of different ages, languages, and cultures who have suffered and continue to suffer the trauma of forced migration.

The great humanitarian crisis of the COVID-19 pandemic has made visible the vulnerability and fragility of us humans, of our limits, and has shown with greater force how the unrepresentable and the unpredictable are presented in our practice.

In this context, migrations have been anticipating a consequence of global capitalism and its failure. The conjunction of inequalities in access to health and education with violence in its various forms added to the climate tragedy of our planet appeals to psychoanalysts not only to contribute our perspective but also to intervene in different scenarios.

Uprooting, xenophobia, and their consequences in the processes of subjectivation are more than evident. This book shows us the possibilities of our discipline to intervene in contexts that go beyond our consulting rooms and institutions.

Vivienne Elton, Vivian B. Pender, Gertraud Schlesinger-Kipp, and Marianne Leuzinger-Bohleber are in charge of several committees and subcommittees of IPA in the community, which started in 2017, and have carried out their task with dedication, conviction, and passion. This new structure, together with the awards given at the last biannual congresses, has made visible the work that many psychoanalysts and candidates are doing in different parts of the world. This book will serve as a stimulus for this work to continue to grow and for analysts with experience and analysts in training to continue to join in.

Not only those who practice it will learn from the experience. The clinical, technical, and theoretical foundations of psychoanalysis will grow and expand only if we pay attention and get involved in the problems of the world we inhabit.

Virginia Ungar, MD, is a training analyst at the Buenos Aires Psychoanalytic Association (APdeBA). She lives and practices in Buenos Aires, Argentina. Virginia specialises in child and adolescent analysis and is the former chair of the IPA's Child and Adolescent Psychoanalysis Committee (COCAP) and of the Committee for Integrated Training. She is the former president of the IPA (2017–2021), receiving the Platinum Konex Award for Psychoanalysis in 2016.

Editorial introduction

Vivienne Elton, Marianne Leuzinger-Bohleber,
Gertraud Schlesinger-Kipp and Vivian B. Pender

Trauma, flight, and migration: a signature of our time

Trauma, flight, and migration have become signatures of our time. Possibly never before in history have this many people been afflicted by persecution, war, and poverty in their native countries and have had to migrate as is the case today. Towards the end of 2021 there were 82.4 million migrants and refugees seeking asylum from their countries of origin in countries far away from war, civil unrest, and economic turmoil. This is an unprecedented number, even greater than the time following World War II. Migration and exile have occurred recently in these huge numbers because of wars in the Middle East, most notably and recently in Syria and Yemen and civil unrest in countries such as Venezuela, in Afghanistan and now in the Ukraine.[1] In addition, there is a dire economic need for many African nationals to continue to seek a better life for themselves and their families. Although there are around 6.5 million Africans who seek migration to Europe yearly, nearly three times as many as in 2008 (2.3 million), there are many more who migrate within Africa to neighbouring countries (22.2 million).

In making journeys of hundreds or thousands of kilometres, many refugees have experienced severe trauma, with violence, kidnaping, trafficking, and separation from their families.

Many migrants are turned back and sent to unsuitable, overcrowded detention camps, where they experience further trauma and danger of death. The numbers of refugees from South to North America and in countries within South America such as from Venezuela and Peru to countries such as Argentina and Chile are escalating.

Migrants and refugees often suffer from mental health problems, having experienced crises caused by dislocation from their homes, with a loss of all that is familiar. This may lead to identity issues, especially in younger migrants. A sense of belonging is crucial in assisting the adjustment of migrants to their new country, no matter what the cause of leaving their homeland.

DOI: 10.4324/9781003203223-1

The crisis of migration may result in personal catastrophe, or creative inner development, with enrichment of the personality. On the one hand, people experience sadness, anxiety, nostalgia, and severe pain of loss; on the other, they carry hope and expectation.

Migration is a potentially traumatic event, with a loss of the containing object, the "motherland." The affected person may experience dissociation, with the host country seen as the holder of all that is good, or alternatively, the original country may contain the good and the host country may become a frightening, unfriendly, and unhelpful place. Nostalgia for what has been lost may be a source of pain in the long term. Alternatively, a loss of good memories may make it difficult to recover from the losses of family, country, and language.

These include losses, both in their countries of origin and en route to their host countries. They have arrived either alone or with their families. If their trauma remains untreated, the traumatic experiences may lead to chronic psychological symptoms or illnesses such as depression, anxiety, or PTSD. The incidence of symptoms is as high as 30%. These refugees suffer from insecurity in their current living conditions and need support and treatment (Akhtar, 2010; Leuzinger-Bohleber & Parens, 2018)

Newcomers may be feared and rejected as the "other," and anxieties can be stirred up by the rhetoric of politicians. However, countries such as Australia, the United States, Canada, Argentina, Israel, and many others, communities have prospered because of successive waves of migrant populations. Migrants have brought enthusiasm, commitment, dedication, and worked hard with hopes of success in their new homelands (Elton, 2019).

Climate catastrophe, global injustice, migration, and pandemics: a fatal alliance

The COVID-19 pandemic has changed our world in a previously unimaginable way within a very short time. Even if there is light at the end of the tunnel in many countries, thanks to vaccinations and falling incidence of severe illness, there will be no going back to the way things were before the pandemic. The longing for normality; for free movement locally, nationally, and internationally; for physical contact and fearless closeness; for carefree encounters; for demonstrations, concerts, and celebrations in public spaces is understandable – but an illusion. We will have to learn to live with globalised dangers such as pandemics.

In many publications and lectures, the sociologist Stephan Lessenich has pointed out the fatal alliance and complex interconnection between a globalised, exploitative economy, climate change, and migration movements. For example, in his book *Neben uns die Sintflut. Externalisierungsgesellschaft und ihr Preis* (2016) *(Beside Us, the Flood. The Externalization Society and Her Prize)*, he describes the mentality of "always more" that not only defines the economics of a globalised capitalism, but also Western democracies. In democracies, too, citizens latently or openly expect a constant improvement in their living conditions, their educational opportunities, their wealth, and so on. This expectation is therefore causally linked to an exploitative economic system that constantly increases injustice within individual societies, but especially in the globalised world. As is well known, this mentality of exploitation is also one of the main reasons for the impending climate catastrophe. Nature shows us the hardly reversible consequences of limitless exploitation. Droughts, floods, storms are now destroying the livelihoods of millions of people around the world, leading to new, warlike conflicts over dwindling resources and inevitably resulting in today's refugee flows (see also Tooze, 2021).

The COVID-19 pandemic has increased social injustice: the gap between the privileged and the underprivileged, the rich and the poor, has widened. The 75 million jobs that will be cut worldwide because of the pandemic disproportionately affect low-skilled workers. The educational losers due to COVID-19 are mainly children from poor families, often with a migration background. Vaccines have almost exclusively benefited the rich countries, Africa is so far an "unvaccinated continent" (ZDF Tagesschau, June 2, 2021).

Stephan Lessenich sketches a bleak picture: if the mentality of "more and more," exploitation and unjust distribution of resources, education, and wealth continues to increase, there will be flight and persecution, and an increasing mass migration. The "black continent" will at some point fight back after a long history of exploitation, starting with colonialism, slavery, and the plundering of mineral and natural resources and ending with the consequences of a climate crisis that it has only marginally contributed to but will have to endure the consequences. "Fortress Europe" will be stormed. Europe will be forced to share its accumulated wealth with the Third World, and its standard of living will fall.

Many of us experienced feelings of extreme helplessness and shame in August 2021 when we saw the images of the desperate people at the airport in Kabul, Afghanistan, attempting to flee the threatening terror regime of the Taliban.

Over the last 20 years, a new Afghan generation has grown up. As they rebuilt their country, they also worked to address the emotional distress that seemed so pervasive in themselves and in the institutions around them. Some became mental health professionals committed to developing a complex national plan to integrate mental health and psychosocial support services into public services from schools, health clinics, and juvenile justice centres to women's NGOS spanning all of Afghanistan's 491 districts, urban and rural. In addition, they worked to develop an Afghan psychology that could effectively address emotional suffering in a cultural context. Their research on curriculum development and the cultural nature of well-being has been published in international journals. As of this writing, many of the Afghan specialists who led this work remain trapped in Afghanistan, under constant threat for their lives.[2] Our colleague, Martha Bragin, accompanied them on this journey and continues to try to find ways to free them. She has described extreme feelings of helplessness, which we as psychoanalysts share in our work with Afghanistan refugees in different countries.

Many of the psychoanalysts who have written chapters for this book will address the profound experience of limitation and loss in the face of pervasive structural violence in the 21st century.

As psychoanalysts, we must ask the pressing question of whether and in what way we, with our specific knowledge of unconscious fantasies and conflicts, can contribute to understanding and dealing with the current situation. This book is dedicated to reflecting on some aspects of this complex, pressing situation.

Psychoanalytical conceptualisation of trauma and migration[3]

In the introduction to their classic book on psychoanalytic migration research titled *Psychoanalysis of the Migration and Exile*, Grinberg and Grinberg (1984) discuss that the topic of migration is as old as the human civilisation, here referring to myths and fairy tales as, for example, the Odyssey. The longing of human beings for new adventure and innovative life perspectives dates back to the roots of mankind as well as the experiences associated with these longings: such as feelings of uprooting, losses, grief, and of being and remaining a foreigner in the new environment – the longing to return to one's own home country. "Homer indicates that the *Odyssey* is about the struggle to get home, or, to use a colloquial expression, it is about Odysseus dying to return home" (Papad opoulos, 2002, p. 11).

Migration, persecution, and flight are also latent topics in the myth of Oedipus, which had been central in the history of psychoanalysis. As is well known, Oedipus was given away by his parents to be killed because the Delphi oracle predicted that he would marry his mother and kill his father. However, the child was saved by a shepherd. As a grown-up "adolescent migrant," he indeed turned into the murderer of his father, Laios: he killed an old man in kind of an adolescent affective outburst because this old man literally stood in his way. He had no idea that this old man was his father. When he was eventually confronted with the unbearable truth, he blinded himself and fled from his home country, Theben. The rest of his miserable life he spent in exile in Kronos.

Female protagonists also, such as Persephone, the loyal wife of Odysseus, or Medea, remind us that migration, flight, and trauma may create existential threats for women and their motherhood. Medea, a priestess and daughter of the demigoddess Hecate and the king Aetes in Colchis, helped Jason to acquire the Golden Fleece, which meant that she had to assist him in killing her brother. Therefore, she had to flee with him. In Corinth, Medea – as a refugee – turned into a foreigner, an archaic witch in the perception of Jason. To ensure that he and their two sons had a permanent refuge, Jason abandoned her and married Creon's daughter Creusa. Medea first became severely suicidal but then remembered that she was a king's daughter. She killed her two sons to take revenge. In her dialogue with Jason at the end of Euripides tragedy, she is filled with simultaneous pain and grief at her children's death but also with the satisfaction of having avenged herself on her husband.

As Leuzinger-Bohleber (2001, 2014) has discussed in several clinical papers, Medea corresponds to central unconscious fantasies of women and their conviction that the dependency of a love object, due to sexual passion and the sometimes traumatic separation from one's own homeland (the mother), may evoke uncontrollable affects and impulses which could result in suicidal and murderous actions even towards one's own children. Traumatic conditions of flight, persecution, and migration contribute to the triggering of such ubiquitous archaic fantasies. Often, one motivation for refugees to leave their country is to save the lives of their children and to guarantee a better future for them. The love and affection for the children is, for many of them, a source of strength and vitality, helping them to survive. Therefore, aggressive fantasies and impulses are particularly hard to cope with for them and often must be denied and split off.

Psychoanalysis, with its knowledge concerning such archaic unconscious fantasies and conflicts, may offer professional help for refugees to understand such difficult psychic processes, particularly in early parenthood (eg, Raphael-Leff and Varvin in this volume).

Many contemporary psychoanalytical authors describe migration and flight as a traumatising event[4] connected with a dramatic loss of one's home, culturally meaningful systems, and a loss of basic feelings of safety in the home culture (Garland et al., 2002; Kogan, 2011; Papadopoulos, 2002; Rickmeyer et al., 2015; Volkan, 2018, Jović, Varvin, and Raphael-Leff in this volume). The process of migration signifies a massive psychic destabilisation and disorganisation because

> there is no place like home. . . . When people lose their homes and become refugees, there is bewilderment, a sense of unreality and of an inexplicable gap because people lose something they were not aware they had in the first place. . . . Whenever the home is lost, all the organizing and containing functions break wide open and there is a possibility of disintegration at all three levels: at the

individual-personal level; at the familial-marital; and at the socio-economic/cultural political levels.

(Papadopoulos, 2002, pp. 9, 18, and 24)

The loss of "the other" who guarantees the psychosocial identity and a basic sense of the self triggers the narcissistic self-regulation. Houzel (1996) introduced the term *psychic envelope* in order to describe the containing function of a group, a family, a culture. For many refugees, particularly for those who had to flee alone without family members, this psychic envelope is missing and leads to a vulnerable psychic state. Luci (2017) characterises this process in refugees as *"losing a psychic skin"*. Just to mention another perspective: the aforementioned psychic and psychosocial processes also might lead to specific inner conflicts and manifest traumatisations. Clinical psychoanalytical studies illustrate that migrants often suffer from severe loyalty conflicts. Having left their families is experienced as an act of aggression and betrayal, a violation of one's ego ideal and superego (Leuzinger-Bohleber, 2016, Bohleber, 2010).

In the host country, migrants maintain the status of a foreigner for a long time. They suffer from the prolonged anxiety and fear of losing one's own personal and cultural identity (Khoshrouy-Sefat, 2007). The ethnopsychoanalyst, Maya Nadig (1986) even talks about a feeling of "social death" in migration. Finally, migration is always connected with separation, loss, and a sense of deserting or being deserted even if migration was not forced but chosen (Volkan, 2018, Jović in this volume).

On the other hand, migration does not always turn into a manifest traumatic experience. The essential role in making it a non-traumatic experience is in allowing it to be psychologically coped with, accepting professional and semiprofessional help in enabling an adequate mourning process. Personality traits prior to the migration as well as the reactions of those who have been left and those who are welcoming the refugees also play an important role. Furthermore, it is important to consider that migration is not just one single act. In the migration process, many factors are intertwined. Factors such as anxiety and psychic pain, when combined, lead to the sustaining negative effects of migration. Kogan, 2011, p. 291). Ilany Kogan mentions five traumatising factors: "1. Separation and loss and, 2011 disruption 2. Loneliness and a feeling of not belonging to anyone 3. Migration as threat of identity 4. Regression or infantilisation as a consequence of migration and 5. Deferred mourning because of migration" (Kogan, 2011).[5]

Preceding traumatising experiences can complicate the mourning processes that are necessary in order to master the migration experience. Volkan (2018) writes in addition: "Without help these people will often mourn forever" (p. 26). It is also well known in clinical surroundings that refugees who have been severely traumatised even before their flight, sometimes suffer from inner persecutory fantasies that make the separation processes from the home country even more difficult for them.

Hence, migration experiences are always a heavy burden, but do not always end in severe traumatisation. As many authors expressed: the short-term and long-term consequences of flight and migration also essentially depend on the conditions in the host country, particularly on the public attitude towards refugees (Geschire, 2009; Varvin, 2016).

Activities of the International Psychoanalytical Association

IPA in the Humanitarian Field Committee: Chair Vivienne Elton

In one of the important innovations of her presidency, Virginia Ungar established a number of new committees in the IPA, developing and investigating work undertaken in the community, including the IPA in the Humanitarian Field Committee. The IPA in the Humanitarian Field Committee includes the Migrants and Refugees and the IPA and the United Nations subcommittees.

Our mandate includes gathering worldwide data about the work of our colleagues and sharing it with our community both within the IPA and with people interested in this work in the humanitarian field.

This book reveals the thinking and work of a small group of the many psychoanalysts who are currently working in the humanitarian field.

It has been inspiring to learn about the endeavours of our psychoanalyst colleagues who are working globally in the humanitarian area, with migrants and refugees, and assisting many groups of people who are in dire need, due to war, famine, poverty, violence, and climate disasters.

We hope to develop and further relationships between psychoanalysts and members of the helping community working in humanitarian organisations and to create networks to enhance an interchange of ideas and experiences and extend our knowledge and theoretical understandings of working in the humanitarian field.

As part of our project, the IPA has offered prizes biennially to the best projects involving the IPA and the community. As a result, we have discovered more members and societies working with migrants and refugees in many innovative and fascinating projects.

It is our mandate to stimulate other analysts to engage in this important field and take their psychoanalytic understanding into the many areas of community life where this can be of help.

The Subcommittee for Migration and Refugees: Chair Gertraud Schlesinger-Kipp

According to the Mid-Year Report of UNHCR Global Trends (2021), the number of people running away from wars, persecutions, and conflicts were over 84 million – a sharp increase from 82,4 million in 2020; 68% of the refugees come from countries such as Syria, Afghanistan, South Sudan, Myanmar, and Venezuela. More than 1,600 refugees died trying to cross the Mediterranean Sea in 2021. Families with children are starving, freezing, and dying at the border between Belarus and Poland, and the EU is only watching this catastrophe.

Since August 2021, after the Western countries left Afghanistan alone to the power of the Taliban there have been many more Afghan refugees and will be in the years to come. We have the moral responsibility to give them secure shelter in our countries.

Acknowledging this as one of the most important worldwide issues, the IPA created the Migration and Refugees committee as a Subcommittee of the IPA and Humanitarian Organisations Committee. Not only does this major issue have an impact on the population but also on the life and practice of analysts who live in countries that are significantly affected by this problem.

The IPA, on the other hand, has the capacity to develop research, therapeutic treatment, and initiatives in the communities, which could foster integration, work with racism, and the violation of human rights as well as improve the treatment of traumatised refugees. The committee is working on mapping the psychoanalytic work done in this area, identifying all existing programs and projects worldwide, finding out where people need help and developing more projects in those areas. We try to promote an interchange between groups working in this area, through sharing experiences, building up common projects, and helping those working in this area.

In addition, various panels on refugees, trauma, and migration have been held at Pre-congress meetings and during the main IPA Congress in London and during the online Vancouver pre-congress and led to an intensive exchange between different groups of psychoanalysts working for refugees and migrants in different countries. The psychoanalytical conceptualisations, understandings, and evaluations of the projects have been very varied and different – hence, the idea arose to publish the papers given in London, in addition to some further contributions in this volume.

The UN sub-committee: Chair Vivian B. Pender

In 1997, the IPA formed its committee on the United Nations, its mandate to bring international issues and concerns to the psychoanalytic profession, with a view to developing a methodology linking individual development to socioeconomic development in the world community. The Committee to the United Nations was founded to make psychoanalysis visible and heard in the United Nations system in general and in the meetings of the Economic and Social Council and its subsidiary bodies and to interact with other non-governmental organisations working with the United Nations system, particularly through the many established NGO (non-governmental organisation) committees of potential interest to the psychoanalytic profession.

The UN system is composed of 193 government missions, hundreds of UN agencies, and over 5,000 non-governmental organisations. By 1998, the IPA had been vetted and officially granted special consultative status by the UN. This designation conferred upon the IPA access to all components of the UN system – a status not ordinarily given to organisations without proof of legitimacy, democracy, and high standards. The UN Universal Declaration of Human Rights highlights the critical importance of peace and security for all humans in the world. As an NGO with special consultative status, the IPA has a responsibility and obligation to contribute to the goals of the UN.

The IPA brings international issues and concerns to the psychoanalytic profession, with a view to developing a methodology linking individual development to socioeconomic development in the world community. The IPA assesses the state of the discipline and practice of psychoanalysis considering such international concerns as conflict prevention and resolution and the effects of prejudice and ethnicity, gender, violence, child abuse, and in general, the promotion of international welfare.

The following are a few examples of the committee's activities relevant to migration.

Xenophobia, racism, and social exclusion are significant factors the committee considered that impact migrants' mental health and sense of well-being. More importantly, xenophobia may be used to victimise large segments of the population by imposing government barriers, decreased funding, legal barriers, and lack of coordination of services. Host communities that were resistant to welcoming refugees were found to have economic, cultural, structural, and safety concerns. These included fear of losing jobs and economic opportunities to migrants, fear of losing or erasing culture due to more diversity, fear of migrants straining social services and infrastructure, and fear of an increase in crime or terrorism and its impact on physical safety. IPA members found it important to assess these issues to aid their work in such communities. Sometimes working with potential messengers such as athletes, celebrities, social media influencers, and migrants themselves to address the positive impact migration can have on communities effected changes in attitudes. Public health services are necessary to attend to basic needs, education, financial support, public awareness, legal aid, social inclusion, and capacity building.

Together with the International Organization for Migration (IOM), a UN subsidiary, the IPA UN Committee has worked with the Global Forum for Migration and Development (GFMD) and the Mayors Mechanism, a platform to ensure meaningful engagement of cities and local governments on balancing migration narratives in countries such as Colombia, Canada, Ecuador, Honduras, Greece, Turkey, Lebanon, and Ghana. The IPA and other non-governmental organisations (NGOs) collectively strategise to negotiate global processes for migration.

The IPA UN Committee participated in research that examined how people's social identities impact their interpretations of intergroup contexts and their experiences while interacting with members of other groups. Understanding how these interactions enhance groups' psychological investment in equality has helped to inform interventions to bridge group differences in the United States, Rwanda, and Bosnia and Herzegovina. The IPA has advocated for the inclusion of psychological research for UN policy. In the United States, the IPA has worked with the Texas Border Collaboration Network to include family mentoring, project development, and outreach to help resettle refugees in neighbourhoods, ignite unity, pride, and dignity through education and advocacy and transition them to self-sufficiency.

Some individuals are smuggled across borders only to be trafficked for labour or commercial sex in the host country. Traffickers prey on these vulnerable people, mostly women and children, who do not have access to human rights mechanisms. However, the IPA UN Committee worked with many NGOs and the US ambassador to Monitor and Combat Trafficking in Persons to advise international governments on protecting victims and survivors. The United States offers a special T-visa for people who have been trafficked. In 2014 the IPA UN Committee presented the trafficking situation at the winter meeting of the American Psychoanalytic Association. It was apparent that many in the audience were naïve to the prevalence of trafficking. Further, although it was found that over 85% of victims had visited a health care professional while in captivity, very few clinicians were aware. In 2015 the committee, together with Weill Cornell Medical College, organised a panel of experts to conduct a half-day training webinar. The experts included a member of Congress, an FBI special agent, a US attorney, an obstetrician-gynaecologist, and four psychoanalysts. One year later, all licensed health care professionals in the state of New York were mandated by law to receive a training course in human trafficking to maintain their license. The training included identification of victims and risk factors, treatment, and referral resources. Reporting mechanisms were also in the process of being organised. This is one remarkable example of how psychoanalysts can work in the community with a coalition.

Aims of this publication

This publication could help to intensify the networking between the different groups to stimulate and enrich each other and learn from our different experiences. In addition, we hope to motivate other colleagues to get involved in the work with refugees and migrants, because we think that psychoanalysis – as a science of the unconscious – has a unique conceptual and clinical contribution to make in understanding the short- and long-term consequences of migration and trauma, as well as in the therapeutic and preventive treatment of them.

Another objective is the exchange between the IPA in the Humanitarian Field committee, the Subcommittee for Migration and Refugees, and the sub-committee for Psychoanalysis and the UN. This volume contains contributions by colleagues from the various committees.

We regard this volume as the first of a collection of reports followed by further publications as well as a database of humanitarian work done world-wide by members and psychoanalysts in training on the IPA website and our new website "An Open Door Review of the IPA in the Humanitarian Field," which will hold more writing about projects in the field. Therefore, this volume has the character of a "work in progress."

Conceptualisation of the volume

Part A of this volume consists of reports of individual projects with refugees and migrants and traumatised poverty-stricken populations from different IPA members and societies. Most of these reports were presented at the IPA Congress in London in 2018. We have complemented them with more reports from other countries.

Part B consists of papers by members of the IPA at the UN committee, thinking about how psychoanalysis and psychoanalytic thinking can be used in the field of human rights and considering their experience of working in the United Nations, with a focus on "The Feminine", the title of the 2018 IPA Congress.

Part A: working with traumatised refugees and migrants

I: Marianne Leuzinger-Bohleber, Gertraud Schlesinger-Kipp, Nora Hettich, in their chapter, "What has clinical psychoanalysis to offer to traumatised refugees? Some experiences during the so-called 'refugee crisis' in Hesse (Germany)" integrate psychoanalytic experiences of two groups working in Hesse (Frankfurt and Kassel). In a short introduction the authors discuss the close connection between climate change, poverty, and war, with migration, flight, and trauma taking up the concept of the Great Regression (Geiselberger), which explains phenomena like extreme societal denials, splitting and threats to democratic structures, xenophobia, nationalism, and populism in many countries. Psychoanalytic considerations of unconscious determinants can usefully complement such sociological analyses. The psychoanalytic knowledge on trauma, flight, and migration formed the basis for the conceptualisation of the pilot project STEP-BY-STEP in the initial-reception centre "Michaelisdorf" 2016/2017

(Leuzinger-Bohleber et al., 2016, 2017). Marianne Leuzinger-Bohleber and Nora Hettich (Part I) describe some of the experiences and the results of the scientific evaluation, which seem to be transferable to other initial-reception facilities, even in other countries. Based on two detailed case studies it is illustrated that – in the sense of SECOND STEPS – longer-term psychoanalytic psychotherapy seems to be quite useful, but only after the refugees have obtained a secure status in the host country, have learned the language, and can earn their living. Only then is it possible to jointly understand the trauma suffered psychoanalytically and *offer some psycho-therapeutic help.*

In Part II, Gertraud Schlesinger-Kipp describes the project of Alexander-Mitscherlich-Institute in Kassel, Germany, where about 25 psychoanalysts and psychotherapists realised a psychosocial and psychotherapeutic approach in an institution for refugees (camp) in Kassel, who are searching for shelter and asylum in Germany. She discusses the limits and chances of sometimes single encounters especially in a situation four years after the initial "welcome" culture in Germany. Today, the right Nazi movement is a great danger for the democratic society. The hate, the threat, and the violence hit the most vulnerable group – the refugees. The psychotherapeutic work with refugees is increasingly thwarted from many sides under this societal split.

II: Annabelle Starck, Željko Čunović, and Rosalba Maccarrone Efhardt: "A quite 'normal' treatment with a refugee in the form of the International Clinic as part of the training outpatient clinic at the Frankfurt Psychoanalytic Institute"

In their contribution, Annabelle Starck, Željko Čunović, and Rosalba Maccarrone Erhardt present psychoanalytic work with refugees in the International Clinic (IC) at the Frankfurt Psychoanalytic Institute (FPI) in Frankfurt am Main. The IC is part of the Psychosozialer Verbund Rhein Main (PSV), in which five organisations with many years of experience in working with trauma, migration, and flight work together. Psychoanalytic therapy and counselling services with and without interpreters offer refugees prompt initial stabilisation and crisis intervention. Some patients also opt for longer and more in-depth treatment. After a presentation of the work of IC (Ž. Čunović and R. Maccarrone Erhardt), Ms Starck, candidate in DPV training, will demonstrate low-frequency psychotherapy with a patient from North Africa. She will focus on the extent to which the training situation additionally influences the constellation of psychotherapy "in threes" – that is, with the support of an interpreter. She will show what necessities dealing with traumatised refugees often are demanded of us. Through reflection in supervision and with oneself, this treatment retains the psychoanalytical character that we care for deeply. Finally, our colleague shows how she was able to help improve the psychological condition of a severely traumatised woman and give her a new perspective on life.

III: Elizabeth Haworth, Lima: "Forced to flee: the experience of Peruvian women in times of political violence"

In this chapter, I discuss a paradox of forced migration in the case of women in Peru: on one hand, it implies an uprooting imposed by external conditions and, on the other, it is also an opportunity for new encounters and an attempt to solve previous conflicts. For women, forced migration involves a strong degree of coercion but, in many cases, also a decision for change and an illusion of improving their lives. In this sense, there is an element of agency that is often overlooked in theoretical discussions on forced migration and in public policies targeted to migrant women.

The sources used are a) the Report by the Commission of Truth and Reconciliation (CTR) submitted in 2002, which collected 12,000 testimonies; b) cases from the Centro de Atención Psicosocial (CAPS), one of the civil society organisations in charge of the legal and psychoanalytical care of cases of torture and political violence; c) a qualitative research study on the object relationships of women who migrated from Ayacucho to Lima when they were children due to the Internal Armed Conflict (IAC), using the TAT. The revision of the sources led us to organise the work around three themes: i) the sudden transition from mothers to heads of household, ii) past and present violence, iii) the transgenerational impact in the daughters of migrants, iv) state reparation policies that interfere with an internal elaboration of the situation.

Though there is an extensive literature on women and forced displacement, we conclude that the influence of IAC in the feminine imaginary has not been fully investigated. In research studies and social movements, we see a split between an image of *brave, empowered women, mothers-fathers*, and *suffering victims*. But women's own decision is not stressed. Finally, the appearance of gangs of adolescent women after the IAC whose violence is pure discharge, without target and the high rate of femicides in Peru are two dramatic events that may have relations with these changes. There is the need to understand the feminine in relation to the masculine, associated with the feminist movements that have been very influential in the country and in the region.

IV: Joan Raphael-Leff: "Perinatal migration: lived experience and intergenerational transmission"

Leaving the motherland is particularly poignant for a childbearing woman. Drawing on 55 years of professional specialisation in reproductive issues, the author's clinical understanding is enhanced by consultative work to perinatal projects on six continents. She engages with both universal commonalities and cultural diversities, focusing on the emotional experiences of pregnant migrants and immigrant mothers, and of the perinatal therapists, counsellors, midwives, and health visitors, or lay practitioners working with them.

The need for personal recognition is at the heart of our human condition. But a migrant can no longer take for granted being known or knowing. This has implications for pregnancy and confidence in mothering.

This chapter draws on my half century of specialisation in reproductive issues. In addition to clinical work and workshops/focus groups with expectant/parents, I have served as consultant to perinatal services in over 40 countries, providing teaching, training and clinical supervision to professional therapists, lay practitioners, counsellors, primary health carers, midwives, health visitors, and so on in groups and/or individually (usually through interpreters). Programmes differ in setting, venue, and content of their provisions from bare minimum to ongoing home visits; from a one-off meeting to ongoing help; before, during and/ or after the birth; from open-ended to theme-based sessions in group, individual, or family sessions; conducted in baby clinics or detention centres; or in home visits to township shacks, city dwellings, or more affluent suburbia. Some projects focus specifically on migrants; others are inclusive, screening all local childbearing women, including those from elsewhere. But in common, these innovative ventures (usually run by non-profit NGOs) aim to reduce emotional distress, while promoting physical safety.

It is noteworthy that cross-cultural work or that in multiethnic societies raises epistemological issues about imposing our own theoretical framework, values, and tacit assumptions on others in the context of language barriers, cultural differences, and hierarchical power structures.

V: Johanna Mendoza Talledo, Lima: "Psicólogos contigo: working with displaced habitants because of a natural disaster"

This chapter gives account of the gestation process of the Contigo Psychologists (Psychologists with You) project (Peru) promoted by the Peruvian Society of Psychoanalysis (SPP) and comprising seven institutions, all of them with a psychoanalytic approach.

In 2017 heavy rains and huaycos caused by the El Niño Costero, a natural phenomenon characterised by the anomalous warming of the sea, led to floods affecting the towns around Lima. A call was made to the members of the SPP and psychoanalytic guidance institutions to propose volunteers to provide group psychological care of people affected in areas near Lima.

One of the affected locations was the town of Barba Blanca, in the province of Huarochirí, in the Sierra of Lima, Peru. The cooperation between neighbouring towns saved the inhabitants of the town, so there were no human losses and the population managed to move to a higher and safer area.

VI: Gilbert Kliman, Los Angeles: "From a trench in the war against children"

When in May 2018 the US government announced an official policy of separating children from asylum-seeking parents, the author rapidly responded. He organised and trained psychoanalysts to provide evaluations suitable for courtroom use for protection of the children. He recommended and is principal clinical expert in a resulting lawsuit against US Immigration and Customs Enforcement and a private jail in which parents and children have been detained. In the process of evaluating over 50 asylum seekers, his psychoanalytic thinking has grappled with the question of what drives human beings and their institutions to destroy others, even children. This endeavour continues the 1915 unsuccessful struggle of Freud and Einstein concerning "Why War?"

VII: Debra Gill: "Suffering from elsewhere: trauma and its transmission"
When treating individuals and families who are unconscious carriers of suffering from elsewhere, psychoanalysis offers an added dimension for listening, silently holding, and eventually coming into contact with intergenerational trauma. Recent literature in the field, particularly the study of forced immigration, the impact of racism, and understanding the experience of "othering" has brought into focus that psychoanalysis has moved too far from human tragedies caused by different legacies of violence stemming from the sociopolitical world. Following a selected review of the literature on trauma and its transmission, this chapter will rely on clinical vignettes of the analytic process where the patient evidenced psychic deadness, mental barriers, and erasure until loss and mourning for parents and in one case, ancestors, could be thought about and experienced. Attention to real and imagined differences in the analytic dyad are discussed in this context.

VIII: Fabio Castriota, Rome: "Psychoanalysis and the drama of refugees in Italy"
In March 2016 the executive of SPI (Italian Psychoanalytical Society) set up the PER Working Group that from the beginning wanted to call itself European Psychoanalysts for Refugees with the intention of making the awareness of the migrant issue deeply affect all of us European colleagues. It requires the development of a thought and a clinical practice capable of dealing with new dimensions of the question of integration and/or coexistence of different needs, cultures, and perspectives.

As for the group (for which Fabio Castriota, vice president of SPI, is responsible) the number of members and candidates who have joined exceeds 100 units, representing all the Italian centres of the SPI.

The group is made up of psychoanalysts who already work throughout Italy, carrying out their activities both directly with migrants and with the operators who deal with them in public and private institutions.

After having surveyed the group's wealth of experience, the scope of the interventions was clarified.

The objectives were defined as follows: i) development of psychoanalytic reflection on migratory events; ii) study and development of the psychoanalytic device to be used to make the work of operators who, in various capacities, deal with the health and safety of migrants sustainable (Balint Groups, clinical supervision of health workers and socio-health-care-cultural mediators, training of the operators).

In this chapter, the experiences and conceptualisations of how to support refugees as psychoanalysts will be discussed.

IX: Anna L Christopoulos, Chrysi Giannoulaki, Nicholas Tzavaras, Athens: "Mourning and issues of identity in the treatment of the refugees in Lesvos"

Mourning is considered to be of critical significance for refugees given their multiple and massive losses – loss of the homeland, language, loved ones, socioeconomic position. Perhaps less obvious is the loss of their identity and all that it encompasses as they are called to "give up" their identity and develop a new one in order to adapt to a new sociopolitical environment. Yet identity is integrally involved in the way the mourning process takes place, as this process is in many ways culturally specific and culturally determined. Unfortunately, specific symbols and rituals with particular cultural meaning are often not considered by the therapeutic environment that views mourning within the Western cultural framework. This impedes the work of mourning and can enhance a resistance to mourning that is often found in traumatised individuals. The significance of the cultural dimensions involved in mourning is evidenced in the psychodynamically oriented treatment of Mr Aasha, a refugee in Lesvos, Greece. The psychoanalytically trained psychiatrist, through reverie and reflection on her own analytic experience, as well as a particular text of Freud, was able to understand the specific cultural dimensions that appeared in the clinical material and thus to respond accordingly. This illustrates one of the challenges faced by clinicians who are called upon to accept the intrusion of the "foreign" and to adapt their own therapeutic identity – their clinical understanding and therapeutic approach – to respond to the intrapsychic needs of refugees.

X: Chrysi Giannoulaki, Athens: "Is psychoanalysis of any help for refugees?"

In December 2016, I was offered a position supervising the team of 57 workers, from the NGO *Doctors of the World* on the island of Lesvos. I had deeply conflicted feelings. On the one hand I felt very enthusiastic as I am a grandchild of immigrant Greeks from Asia Minor. At the same time, I was very frightened as the work outside my private practice, and any organised mental health setting seemed very foreign to me. This reminded me the Freudian issue of *unheimlich,* which leads me to recognise the need for a "motherland," a place to belong to, which is so crucial for any refugee. At the same time, I also felt deeply ashamed to talk about this decision with my colleagues: how would I answer to their questions about the setting? I began to feel as an immigrant in my own psychoanalytic country! I decided to accept the position. However, I then found that the psychoanalytically oriented supervision I offered was met with very controversial feelings not only among the psychoanalysts but even by the group of workers of the *Doctors of the World*. They denied the utility of the supervision, and they expressed the wish for me to provide more concrete services such as psychiatric care for the refugees – there was only one psychiatrist in the hospital of Lesvos who failed to meet the need of evaluating even urgent psychiatric problems. I agreed to their request. During the meeting with the refugees, the case workers soon began to appreciate the psychoanalytical approach, as it led to a better understanding of the refugees' traumatic situation. In this chapter, I will try to present some aspects of the interactions between refugees, colleagues, and myself, which led me to consider significant aspects of transference and countertransference phenomena. Of particular importance is the need to detect our own racism towards the refugees, which is frequently hidden under the underestimation of their own values and of their own identity crisis during their migration.

XI: Vladimir Jović, Belgrade: "Schizoid mechanisms in posttraumatic states"

The main aim of this chapter is to illustrate how psychological trauma related to war, torture, and exile can lead to severe pathology that is based on schizoid mechanisms – that is, splitting of larger parts of the self and massive projective identifications due to the impaired process of symbolisation. Immediate impact of trauma is overwhelming anxiety which can be said to be unbounded from a neutralised state in previously healthy individuals. Current traumatic event(s) and affects related to it at first are not represented and can be unobservable until, and if, the integration of traumatic experience becomes inevitable. What can follow in the positive line of development is the process of reintegration, which is usually accompanied by depressive crises and mourning; resolution can be achieved if a person is able to integrate previously non-represented, unconscious experience and affects into his or her personal biographical narrative. In chronic cases we can observe mechanisms which are aimed at prevention of integration of those affects, which keeps them in a raw, overwhelming, and extremely painful form, that lead to behaviour and strategies usually seen in posttraumatic pathology, such as social isolation, restriction of affect, detachment from others, substance abuse, psychosomatic disorders, and so on. While all this has been described before, we believe that it is important to place and recognise these mechanisms in refugee populations that have huge numbers of victims of torture and severe abuse and to contrast it to the simple and mechanistic model of posttraumatic stress disorder which is based on the notion of "traumatic memory" and preassumed pathological mechanisms related to it. In that sense theoretical frameworks are illustrated with short clinical vignettes.

XII: Sverre Varvin, Oslo: "Long-term psychoanalytic treatments with traumatised refugees"

There is increasing evidence that psychoanalytic therapies are helpful for traumatised persons in comprehensive ways in that this approach may help address crucial areas in the clinical presentation of complex traumatisation (complex PTSD) that are not targeted by other current empirically supported treatments (which, of course, may be helpful in their way (eg, CBT and EMDR)). Many refugees have experienced extreme traumatisation both before and during flight and the living conditions in arrival countries are increasingly difficult for many.

Refugees and asylum seekers have in addition to psychic suffering related to traumatisation often problems related to acculturation, family problems, economic problems, and so forth.

Psychotherapy and rehabilitation must then go hand in hand.

Psychoanalytic therapy may be the best treatment approach for many, as it has a historical perspective and works with problems related to the self and self-esteem, enhancing the ability to resolve reactions to trauma through improved reflective functioning, and it aims at internalisation of more secure inner working models of relationships. A further focus is work on improving social functioning. Finally, and this is increasingly substantiated in several studies, psychodynamic psychotherapy also for traumatised patients, tends to result in continued improvement after treatment ends.

In this chapter, I will present the background for psychoanalytic psychotherapy with traumatised refugees. I will underline the need for a long-term approach (lasting more than one year) and present material from refugee patients in psychotherapy.

XIII: Barbara Saegesser; Basel: "Fifteen years of psychoanalytical fieldwork in Eastern African cities"

This paper will describe some of the important issues I have understood from my 15 years of psychoanalytical fieldwork. Beginning in Alexandria and ending at the Indian Ocean, this work spanned a distance of 13,000 km.

I worked in a psychoanalytically informed way with refugees and migrants who have suffered and overcome many ordeals during their fight and flight for survival.

I will refer to refugees from Alexandria (Egypt), Khartoum (Sudan), Addis Ababa and Hawassa (Ethiopia), Djibouti, Kampala (Uganda) and Zanzibar (Tanzania). All these refugees have a similar background to refugees from Eritrea. In Eritrea there was a massive impact from the totalitarian regime, which often provoked specific anxieties and paranoid reactions (in European terms and meaning, although those terms were not the terms understood by the refugees themselves). In Somalia refugees suffered from intense anxiety reactions due mainly to the deadly actions by Al-Shabaab, a terrorist organisation. The same anxiety and paranoid reactions also characterised refugees from Zaire and the Central African Republic.

Refugees from *Eastern Africa* – the poorest part of the dark continent – are, in a cultural, ethnic, and religious way, quite *different* to *refugees* from *Western African* countries.

XIV: David Morgan, London: "The return of the oppressed, the birth of the other, and collective Western guilt"

Entire societies continue to function at a paranoid-schizoid level, risking splits and projections that can only dangerously reduce the safety of the world. I feel that the ethics of migration involve bringing about an awareness of collective guilt in the West that we wish to obviate by locating it outside ourselves.

For Winnicott, the human capacity for a sense of guilt is indicative of individual emotional growth:

> A defective sense of guilt is not linked to intellectual capacity or incapacity but rather the capacity for guilt is linked to the tolerance of ambivalence within the self. In successful analyses of individuals oppressed by guilt, there is a lessening of guilt, though for some the source of guilt cannot be reached, and for those individuals who feel that they are not able to explain this, it can make for a feeling of madness. I think this can also pertain at the societal level.
>
> (Winnicott, 1959, p. 44).

There are many reasons why people migrate, and the author makes some observations about migration to provide an ethical perspective around this emotive issue. He suggests that the migrant is a repository of our own fears, carrying a reminder of Western hegemony and the dreaded retaliation or insight it could bring about. We can experience these reminders as persecuting because they remind us of aspects of our cultural history that we choose to turn a blind eye to.

People migrate owing to a need to survive, to find food, and to avoid danger and death by moving towards opportunities for life that many of us here, through luck and, arguably, an aggressive foreign policy, possess. With the history of privilege many of us from the developed West have benefited from, we can feel we are the beneficiaries of the Lottery of Life, and as winners of the global quasi "Hunger Games" we live in, we are bound to get missives from the oppressed about the injustice of this lottery.

XV: Maya Nadig, Bremen: "On a psychoanalytic attitude towards the culturally and psychologically unknown and its significance for psychoanalytic work with refugees and migrants"

Nadig uses the ethnopsychoanalytic method to understand psychodynamic processes between culturally different partners in analytic work and shows how the psychodynamics between people of different cultures can be viewed and understood. Four examples illustrate the problems of a psychanalytical position in transcultural situations or settings. (i) Field research with the Mosuo: investigating the socialisation of the Mosuo, a matrilineal society without marriage in Southern China, whose members live and produce in large households with maternal blood relatives, she found that their seemingly strange behaviour is indirectly adjusted to the existing living conditions. An inconsiderate recourse to psychoanalytical categories, however, would result in a judgemental, inadequate interpretation of the forms of relationship and their unconscious meaning. (ii) The second example explains the method of ethnopsychoanalytic interpretation workshop. (iii) Then there are theoretical reflections on trauma as well as on real and psychological homelessness. (iv) The last example is a case study about the psychoanalytic process with a patient from a foreign culture. Consequences are the differentiated handling of one's own countertransference, which must be based on different views to the "other" and a multi-perspective approach to the functioning of the unconscious in the foreign culture. It is just on the basis of such processes of self-and-other-reflexivity that one gets to know and understand that assumptions about individual undesirable developments or supposed "neuroses" in the others can be made only as hypotheses and only considering the context of the culture of the other.

Part B: Psychoanalysis and the UN

XVI: Laura Ravaioli, Rome: "Advocating Psychoanalysis at the UN".

The mission of a psychoanalyst at the United Nations is making psychoanalysis visible and heard in the United Nations system, raising the attention of the institutions and other NGOs on mental health, and creating links. In the conferences, IPA is introduced as an association of mental health experts involved in the therapies of the traumatised victims, in the training of health workers, and in outreach initiatives that help to address psychological suffering in the community and identify small- and large-group dynamics correlated to sociopolitical issues. The author shares her experience as a member of the IPA Subcommittee for the UN and includes some reflections about the equilibrium between the masculine and the feminine, essential to overcome divisions and a passive condition of delegating responsibilities and distrust towards institutions. She also reflects on the value of freedom – both intrapsychic and interpersonal – strongly connected to psychoanalysis and migration.

XVII: Paola Amendoeira, Brazil: "The psychoanalyst, psychoanalysis, and human rights: a perspective that instigates us"

What is the territory and size of psychoanalysis? How can it expand, and where does it shrink? At current times, it has been common for us to observe a rescue of Freudian texts considered the social ones.

Psychoanalysts find themselves in a situation of a disturbing uncanniness. Feeling sometimes invited, other times summoned, either internally or externally, to contribute and collaborate to the construction of a space where thoughts can be thought. Through the expansion of the clinic, we can once more observe the "couch starting to move around," reaffirming the commitment to the defence and protection of human rights.

XVIII: Sargam Jain, New York: "The right to stay in place"
The United Nations was created in 1945, after World War II, to ensure cooperation between nations and to act as a peacekeeping body. Over time, it evolved to also set a global progress agenda for its member nations. This agenda primarily targets the material conditions of human life. Interestingly, it does this through prescribing minimum acceptable standards of a home that allows for the well-being of the family that dwells within. However, the United Nations, following the bias of economists, does not consider the labour, primarily performed by mothers, that sustaining such a home requires.

The material conditions of human life are also, in a way, the British psychoanalyst Donald Winnicott's concern. As he notes, a good-enough mother is responsible for a reasonable level of emotional attunement to her child *as well as* maintaining a facilitating environment *in which* this can occur. As psychoanalysts, we focus on the former. But what about the latter? There is scant psychoanalytic research and writing on the function of the physical environment in psychological development.

The role of maternal labour in the production of home life is thus ignored. In this chapter, I speculate that this intellectual neglect is due to the function of *abjection*. Julia Kristeva describes this unconscious mental operation as a defence against the horror of the maternal body and mind, to which we were all once merged. Because home is a symbol of an enveloping maternal body, it cannot be acknowledged by a patriarchal social and economic order.

Women primarily, especially in developing and postcolonial countries where gender roles remain rigid, perform this unvalued maternal labour. However, in the ancient mythology of these places lies rich evidence that the world was not always so. A precolonial sociopolitical order may have once existed that recognised the centrality of the home, as opposed to the current focus on labour performed outside of it (in markets and factories, for example). I argue that a return to this model would strengthen the drive to ameliorate global poverty, in addition to healing the wounds created by the trauma of the colonial experience.

Notes

1 The manuscript of this book was delivered to the publisher before February 24, 2022. At that time, we all did not want to believe that a new terrible war would take place on European soil. Putin's brutal war has forced another 6.5 million people to flee and brought great suffering to millions more.

2 Associate Professor Martha Bragin wrote this paragraph about her experience of working with colleagues in Afghanistan.
3 The following section is based on Leuzinger-Bohleber and Hettich (2018).
4 In this volume, following Bohleber (2010), we are using a narrow concept of "trauma." "Trauma," a sudden, unforeseen, extreme experience, usually associated with life threat and fear of death, breaks through the natural protection against stimuli. The ego is exposed to a feeling of extreme powerlessness and its inability to control or cope with the situation. It is flooded with panic and extreme physiological reactions. This experience results in a state of psychological and physiological shock. The traumatic experience also destroys the empathic shield that forms the internalised primary object, destroying confidence in the continued presence of good objects and the expectability of human empathy. In trauma, the internal good object falls silent as an empathic mediator between self and environment (see also Leuzinger-Bohleber, Hettich & Schlesinger-Kipp and Varvin in this volume).
5 In the research project FIRST STEPS, the Sigmund-Freud-Institut, in cooperation with the Anna-Freud-Institut, has investigated more than 1,000 mothers and families that migrated to Germany. Three hundred of them participated in intensive psychoanalytic prevention groups for more than three years in Frankfurt and Berlin. The psychoanalytically oriented groups have been very helpful and were often able to prevent migration from turning into a severely traumatising event (Leuzinger-Bohleber & Lebiger-Vogel, 2016).

References

Akhtar, S. (2010). *Immigration and acculturation: Mourning, adaptation, and the next generation*. New York: Jason Aronson.
Bohleber, W. (2010). *Destructiveness, intersubjectivity and trauma: The identity crisis of modern psychoanalysis*. London: Karnac Books.
Elton, V (2019, July). Presentation at IPA conference: The feminine: 'Introduction to the migration and refugees committee in the international psychoanalytical association'. In *Trauma, flight and migration: Contemporary threads to the feminine*. London.
Garland, C., Hume, F., & Majid, S. (2002). Remaking connections: Refugees and the development of 'emotional capital' in therapy groups. *Psychoanal. Psychother, 16*(3), 197–214.
Geschire, P. (2009): *The perils of belonging, Autochthony, citizenship, and exclusion in Africa and Europe*. Chicago: The University of Chicago Press.
Grinberg, L., & Grinberg, R. (1984). *Psychoanalytic perspectives on migration and exile*. New Haven, CT: Macmillan and Yale University Press.
Houzel, D. (1996). The family envelope and what happens when it is torn. *International Journal of Psychoanalysis, 77*, 901–912.
Khoshrouy-Sefat, H. (2007). Migration und seelische Krankheit: Analytische Psychotherapie mit Migranten aus traditionsgeleiteten Gesellschaften-speziell aus dem Iran. *Zeitschrift für Individualpsychologie, 32*(3), 245–264.
Kogan, I. (2011). *Mit der Trauer kämpfen: Schmerz und Trauer in der Psychotherapie traumatisierter Menschen*. Stuttgart: Klett-Cotta.
Lessenich, S. (2016). *Neben uns die Sintflut. Die Externalisierungsgesellschaft und ihr Preis*. München: Hanser Verlag.

Leuzinger-Bohleber, M. (2001). The 'Medea fantasy': An unconscious determinant of psychogenic sterility. *International Journal of Psychoanalysis, 82*, 323–345.

Leuzinger-Bohleber, M. (2014). 'Out-reaching psychoanalysis': A contribution to early prevention for 'child-at-risk'? In R. N. Emde & M. Leuzinger-Bohleber (Eds.), *Early parenting and prevention of disorder: Psychoanalytic research at interdisciplinary frontiers* (pp. 20–49). London: Karnac Books.

Leuzinger-Bohleber, M. (2016). From free speech to ISY-pathological regression of some traumatized adolescents from a migrant background in Germany. *International Journal of Applied Psychoanalytic Studies, 13*(3), 213–223.

Leuzinger-Bohleber, M., & Lebiger-Vogel, J. (2016). *Migration, frühe Elternschaft und die Weitergabe von Traumatisierungen – Das Integrationsprojekt "Erste Schritte".* Stuttgart: Klett-Cotta.

Leuzinger-Bohleber, M., & Parens, H. (2018). Editorial to the special issue on trauma, flight and migration. *International Journal of Applied Psychoanalytic Studies.* doi:10.1002/aps.1584.

Leuzinger-Bohleber, M., Rickmeyer, C., Tahiri, M., & Hettich, N. (2016). Special communication. What can psychoanalysis contribute to the current refugee crisis? Preliminary reports from STEP-BY-STEP: A psychoanalytic pilot project for supporting refugees in a "first reception camp" and crisis interventions with traumatized refugees. *International Journal of Psychoanalysis, 11*, 1–17.

Leuzinger-Bohleber, M., Tahiri, M., & Hettich, N. (2017). STEP-BY-STEP. *Psychotherapeut, 62*(4), 341–347.

Luci, M. (2017). Disintegration of the self and the regeneration of 'psychic skin' in the treatment of traumatized refugees. *Journal of Analytical Psychology, 62*(2), 227–246.

Nadig, M. (1986). Die verborgene Kultur der Frau. In *Ethnopsychoanalytische Gespräche mit Bäuerinnen in Mexiko.* Frankfurt am Main: Suhrkamp.

Papadopoulos, R. (Ed.). (2002). *Therapeutic care for refugees: No place like home.* London: Karnac Books.

Rickmeyer C., Lebiger-Vogel J., Busse A., Fritzemeyer K., Burkhardt-Mußmann C., & Leuzinger-Bohleber, M. (2015). Early motherhood in migration: A first report from FIRST STEPS – An integration project for infants with an immigrant background. *Journal of Pregnancy and Child Health, 2*, 147.1

Tooze, A. (2021). *How covid shook the world economy.* New York: Viking.

UNHCR Global Trends. (2021). *UNHCR mid-year-report 2021.* Retrieved from www.unhcr.org/mid-year-trends.html

Varvin, S. (2016). Unsere Beziehung zu Flüchtlingen: zwischen Mitgefühl und Dehumanisierung. *Bulletin of the European Psychoanalytical Federation, 71*, S11–S30.

Volkan, V. D. (2018). Immigrants and Winnicott, D. W. (1986). 10. Transitional objects and transitional phenomena: A study of the first not-me. *Essential Papers on Object Relations, 254*.

Winnicott, D. W. (1959). Psycho-analysis and the sense of guilt. In L. Caldwell & H. Taylor Robinson (Eds.), *The collected works of D.W. Winnicott, Volume 5, 1955–1959.* Oxford: Oxford University Press.

Part A

Psychoanalytical projects "off the couch"

Some examples

1 What has clinical psychoanalysis to offer to traumatised refugees? Some experiences during the so-called "refugee crisis" in Hesse (Germany)

Part I: the STEP-BY-STEP project, Part II: psychoanalytic treatments of refugees in Kassel

Marianne Leuzinger-Bohleber, Gertraud Schlesinger-Kipp, and Nora Hettich

> *We have lost our language and with it the naturalness of our reactions.*
> (Hanna Arendt in: *We Refugees*)

Part I

Trauma, flight, migration, and the "great regression": some introductory remarks

Dealing with traumatised refugees and migrants has become one of the most pressing topics of our world today, especially because it is, as mentioned in the editorial introduction, inextricably linked to the global threat of the climate catastrophe due to the economic and human attitude of greed and exploitation. The resulting destruction of economic livelihoods and the struggle for resources, combined with the diffuse feeling of inscrutable international dependencies, are central causes of armed conflicts, the so-called poverty migration, and the "Great Regression" (Geiselberger, 2017) that has led to a worldwide increase in nationalism, fundamentalism, and populist authoritarianism (Appadurai, 2013). We are experiencing a new shock to Western societies – a social, political, and cultural *"malaise of discomfort"* (Löwenthal, 1990). Donald Trump, but also other populist and authoritarian leaders like Recep Tayyip Erdoğan, Viktor Orbán, or Andrzej Duda, embody in many respects the negation of how the Western

DOI: 10.4324/9781003203223-3

world describes itself: as societies of self-control in which the forces of cultural progress are at home, promoting enlightenment, equality, and social integration.

> Something has slipped in these societies, they are shaken in their self-image: something raw and furious has now entered the political public sphere, it is shamelessly hated, dangerous feelings, fantasies of violence and even desires to kill are frivolously articulated.
>
> (Nachtwey, 2017, p. 215, translation MLB)

The sociologist Oliver Nachtwey (2017) discusses the complex interdependencies of individual and collective experiences of violence in his analyses of the "process of de-civilization" (depletion of civilisation). Nachtway refers to the *Dialectics of the Enlightenment (Dialektik der Aufklärung)* by Max Horkheimer and Theodor W. Adorno on the one hand and to Norbert Elias's theory of *the Civilizing Process (Prozess der Zivilisation)* on the other hand. It is important for us as psychoanalysts to remember that the most important starting point for all these authors was Sigmund Freud's assumption that the development of culture goes hand in hand with a sublimation of impulses so that external constraints on individuals eventually turn into self-imposed constraints. Therefore, according to Horkheimer and Adorno, a rationalised ("enlightened") world also represents a world of anonymised domination which entails the danger of breakthroughs of drives and affects, of barbarism, and the breakdown of civilisation. "Instead of entering into a truly human state, they fear humanity could sink into a new kind of barbarism" (Nachtwey, 2017, p. 219, translation, the authors). Such processes can be observed in many phenomena today in connection with the so-called refugee crisis.

The French sociologist and philosopher Bruno Latour (2017) discusses a frightening, radical hypothesis: namely, that the elites in various Western countries have certainly perceived the coming climate catastrophe since the 1990s but have not drawn from it what we consider to be the desirable conclusion that everything has to be done to save the threatened planet for all of us.

> Rather, they concluded two other things from it, and these ultimately led to King Ubu's entry into the White House: Yes, the return of the earth will certainly cost its prize, but *it will not be us* who pay for it, *but the others*. Moreover, we will simply *deny the undeniable existence of the new climate regime.*

If this hypothesis is correct, we have found the key to understand three developments: what has been known since the 1980s as "deregulation" and "social dismantling"; the "negationism" that has been used since 2000 to confront climate catastrophe; and, finally, the dizzying rise in inequality that we have seen in the last 40 years.

All three developments are part of one and the same phenomenon:

> [T]he elites realized this existential threat by climate change and thus developed the conviction that there cannot be a common future for everyone. Thus, they decided to throw off the ballast of solidarity (hence deregulation) and began to build a kind of golden fortress for the few percent who were supposed to be drawn out of the affair (hence the explosion of inequalities), and last but not least they understood that they could only conceal the bland egoism expressed in such a flight by simply negating the cause of this flight (hence the denial of climate change).
>
> (Latour, 2017, pp. 141–142)

These processes are described also by other authors in the volume *The Great Regression. An International Debate on the Spiritual Situation of Time* (translation by the authors), as an existential threat to Western democracies and human rights.

Psychoanalysis, as a science of the unconscious and human psychodynamics, may complement these sociological analyses and deepen them by unconscious dimensions towards an interdisciplinary understanding of these highly threatening destructive processes that are always mainly related to irrational factors (Akhtar, 2010; Kristeva, 1990; Leuzinger-Bohleber et al., 2016; Volkan, 2018).

As, for example, Bohleber (2010) elaborates, particularly in antisemitism, and in an analogous manner in islamophobia as well as in xenophobia and the violence against migrants and refugees (also connected, as just mentioned with the climate disaster), ubiquitous unconscious phantasy systems are triggered. The foreigner evokes the "phantasma" of "purity" – a narcissistic phantasy of merging with the primary object (Verschmelzungsphantasie), which is always evoked by nationalistic feelings and thinking. According to this phantasma, the foreigner – by his presence – pollutes the "pure idyll" of the homeland, the "father" or "motherland," the nation. Another archaic phantasy is built on early sibling rivalry and envy: the foreigner is experienced as a greedy, voracious intruder who takes away jobs, prosperity, and social welfare and sucks out the "German," the "American," and so on. One's own failure, loss of job, poverty, and all personal misery are unconsciously ascribed to the "other" (i.e., the foreigner) (Leuzinger-Bohleber, 2016).

Another reason for the conflicted and hostile, prejudicial reactions to refugees lies in the fact that refugees fleeing war also evoke unconscious associations linked to "trauma" (Parens, 2014); in other words, extreme experiences that expose the self to fear of death, helplessness, and powerlessness inundate the self in such a way that "basic trust" (Erikson, 1959) in helpful love objects and an actively reliant self is lost (see also the concept of epistemic trust (Fonagy et al., 2019)). The biologically rooted flight impulse is one of the ubiquitous reactions to the perception of trauma and traumatised persons. It is the impulse to look away, to deny, and to turn a blind eye (John Steiner) to the unbearable.

We need to reflect and to counteract this impulse, in order to be able to empathise with traumatised refugees and immigrants and to offer them "a little of that human touch" (Bruce Springsteen). We think that all the authors of this volume – as well as the members of the Committee of IPA in the Humanitarian Field and its Subcommittee for Refugees and Migration – are trying to get involved in exactly this direction, even if this can only be a drop in the ocean.

The STEP-BY-STEP- project, reflecting on some experiences of clinical work with traumatised refugees (Part I) (Marianne Leuzinger-Bohleber, Nora Hettich)

What does psychoanalysis as a science of the unconscious, in which especially individual and cultural fantasies and conflicts have been kept, have to offer to the understanding and the therapeutic treatment of traumatised refugees?

This question leads us again and again into extreme feelings of helplessness and insufficiency, which individually probably can only be coped with by fantasies of omnipotence or other primitive defence mechanisms, like denial, splitting, fragmentation, or projective identification. Therefore, we all need to dialogue with colleagues to be able to think together about the chances, but also the limits of psychoanalytic activities or therapeutic offers to refugees on a mature mental level – for example, in order to cope with one's own ambivalent feelings in the countertransference as well as with the recurring experiences of being overfloated by panic and death-anxiety trying to empathise with the unbearable of trauma which our refugee patients had gone through (Leuzinger-Bohleber et al., 2016).

We collected our psychoanalytic experiences with refugees mostly in the frame of the project "STEP-BY-STEP,"[1] which we would like to introduce only very briefly in this chapter, since it has been published in the meantime and is also available in an impressive film by Rose Palmer www.refugeesfilmfest.com. In addition, Marianne Leuzinger-Bohleber and Gertraud Schlesinger-Kipp have reported on it in podcasts (see IPA website)

Summary of the STEP-BY-STEP project

At the height of the so-called refugee crisis in October 2015, the Hessian Ministry for Social Affairs approached M. Leuzinger-Bohleber as the then director of the Sigmund-Freud-Institute in Frankfurt and asked her to design a concept for the care of traumatised refugees in an initial-reception facility based on her years of experience with psychoanalytically based prevention projects. A corresponding research proposal, together with the educational scientist Sabine Andresen, was approved. The project was carried out in the initial centre "Michaelisdorf" (Michaelis-Village) in Darmstadt in 2016 and 2017. We had a team of about 40 young psychology students and 20 students of educational sciences as well as around 10 experienced psychoanalysts as supervisors, therapists in the village, and so on. The number of refugees in the village fluctuated between 800 (in October 2015) and around 250 (in April 2017). The project was scientifically evaluated, which led to the establishment of three Psychosocial Centres in Hesse, which – after the FIRST STEPS in "Michaelisdorf" – continue to care for refugees in the sense of SECOND STEPS until this day.

To summarise, the most important experiences which could be of interest for other initial-reception centres for refugees:

As part of the STEP-BY-STEP model project, refugees and especially those who have experienced trauma were cared for from the very beginning. In close cooperation with the professional and volunteer teams in the "Michaelisdorf," an attempt was made to offer the refugees initial security and protection through a stable environment as well as reliable, interpersonal experiences in order to reduce the risk of reactivation or re-traumatisation. This proved to be helpful both for the psychological and psychosocial situation of the refugees in the initial-reception facility and for their later readiness to integrate into the host country.

STEP-BY-STEP was well received by the refugees and those working in "Michaelisdorf." The individual offers were based on psychoanalytical and interdisciplinary trauma research on the one hand and social pedagogical concepts for the care of refugee children and adolescents on the other. They proved to be suitable for supporting the refugees and were well implemented in everyday life.

The following concepts, experiences, and results of STEP-BY-STEP have proven helpful and could also be considered in implementations in other initial-reception facilities for refugees:

a) *The close and well-structured cooperation of* psychotherapeutic, medical, social, and educational *experts from the local networks with the professional and volunteer teams in the initial-reception centre.*

b) The *creation of secure and reliable everyday structures* through transparent information on procedures and offers for refugees ("weekly plan"), which is conveyed to them immediately in the first conversation after their arrival.

c) Together with the teams onsite, STEP-BY-STEP tried to contribute to an *atmosphere of interpersonal encounters* as well as empathy for the "unimaginable, what people can do to people."

d) *Alternative relationship experiences were offered that* strengthened the refugees' resilience. Weekly case discussions, team supervisions of the various professional groups and volunteers, and training sessions proved to be helpful in achieving the goals of STEP-BY-STEP.

e) The attitude of *"giving and taking"* (every refugee of any age should "get something" in "Michaelisdorf" for at least two hours a day, but also "give something" to the community for at least two hours themselves) has proven important in returning the refugees from an experience of passivity to active action. In addition, they regained their human dignity to some extent when they were recognised in their specific refugee fate, but also in their personality traits and abilities and were able to contribute these, for example, as translators, educators, craftsmen, artists, and so on to the community in "Michaelisdorf."

f) Cooperation of professional teams and (local) psychotherapeutic trauma experts to carry out an *initial screening for particularly traumatised persons* within the framework of weekly consultation hours in order to provide them – in the sense of FIRST STEPS – with the acute help they need already in the initial-reception facility and to initiate SECOND STEPS in order to enable longer-term professional help after the transfer to permanent accommodation near the initial facilities.

g) *Personal mentorships, supervised by experts in the initial-facility environment* (such as the University of Applied Sciences in Darmstadt) to help students and other particularly vulnerable refugees make the transition from the initial-reception facility to long-term housing.

Clinical psychoanalytic work within an initial-reception centre

In four modules of the STEP-BY-STEP project clinical psychoanalytical work was offered by experienced psychoanalysts: i) in a weekly psychoanalytic-psychosocial consultation hour, ii) a therapeutic painting group for children, iii) in a FRIST STEPS groups for pregnant women and mothers with infants, and iv) in groups for adolescents. We have described all these offers in detail in other publications – for example, in Leuzinger-Bohleber and Hettich (2018). A detailed examination of the experiences of adolescent refugees during their initial time in Germany and a review about psychosocial interventions offered to adolescent refugees after their arrival in a host country can be found in the articles of the cumulative dissertation of Nora Hettich, which was based on the STEP-BY-STEP project (Hettich, in review; Hettich et al., 2020; Hettich & Meurs, 2021). In the frame of this chapter, we just want to refer to the following.

The weekly psychoanalytic-psychosocial consultation hour

In an initial-reception centre for refugees, it is highly important to be able to recognise severely traumatised people and provide first steps of helping in the form of mental and psychosocial emergency aid. STEP-BY-STEP is based on the psychoanalytic as well as on the interdisciplinary trauma research.

Box 1.1   A psychoanalytic definition of traumatisation

During a traumatic experience the natural protection against over-whelming stimulus is destroyed because of a sudden, unforeseeable and extreme experience causing mortal danger and fear of death. The self is exposed to a feeling of extreme powerlessness and the inability to control or manage the situation. It is flooded with panic and extreme physiological reactions leading to a psychological and physiological state of shock. The traumatic experience destroys the empathic shield that the internalized relationship subjects (primary objects) form. Moreover, it destroys the confidence on the continued presence of good relationships and the expectation of human empathy. In the trauma, the memory of inner good persons (good inner objects) as empathic mediators between self and environment falls silent. These processes are connected with an extreme loss of the basic feeling of one's self-agency which has severe short-term and long-term consequences.

(Bohleber, 2010; Leuzinger-Bohleber, 2015)

During specific trainings, the weekly case conferences, and team supervisions, all medical and pedagogic professionals of the "Michaelisdorf" as well as the team members of STEP-BY-STEP got schooled to recognise traumatised refugees.[2] Based on corresponding everyday observations (or specific information from the refugees themselves), vulnerable persons were presented in the weekly psychosocial consultation hour. Particularly traumatised people received several psychoanalytically oriented crisis interventions, often in close collaboration with the medical and social team of the "Michaelisdorf" (Leuzinger-Bohleber et al., 2017). If necessary, the client also got medication in addition to the crisis interventions (subscribed by the psychiatric colleagues). The consultations were documented systematically considering the data protection carefully. Subsequently, all information was discussed during the weekly case conferences in order to jointly initiate "first steps" in the initial-reception centre. Furthermore, "second steps" (medical, psychotherapeutic, psychosocial, educational care) were initiated to support traumatised persons after the transfer to long-term accommodation in the Darmstadt or the Frankfurt area.

Figure 1.1 shows the flowchart of this process.

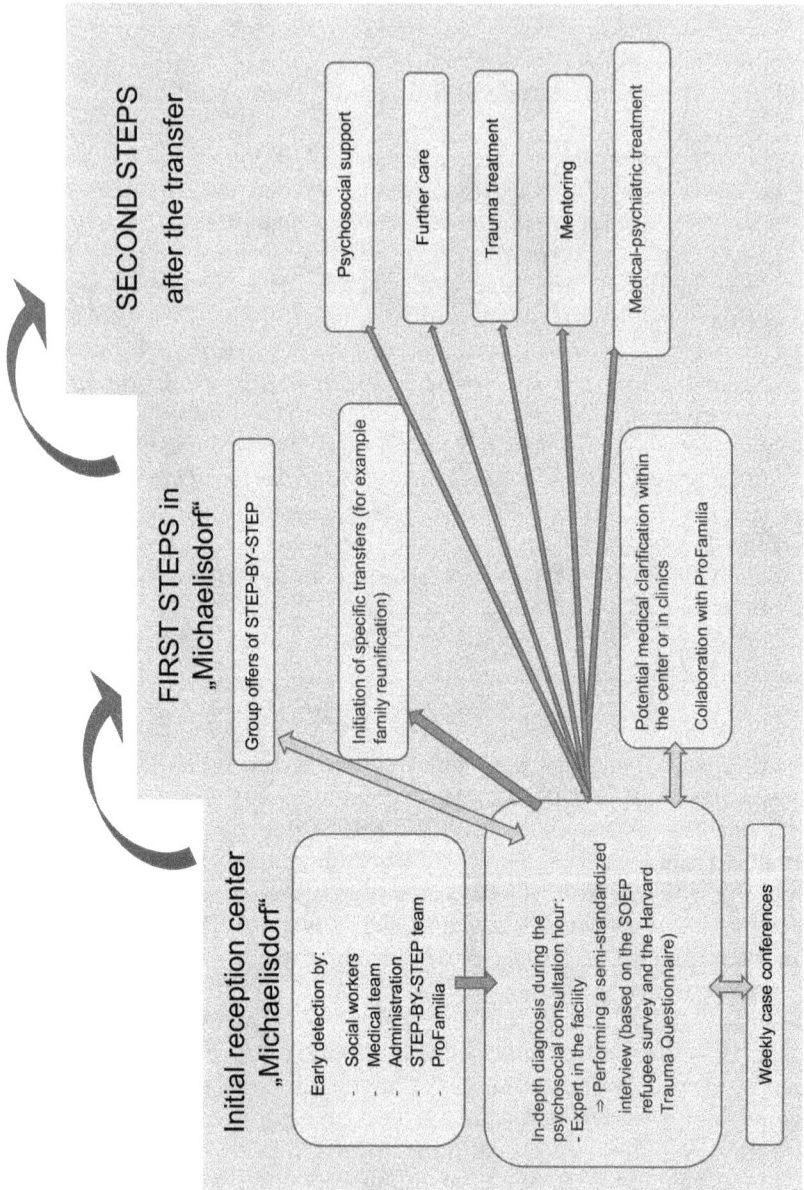

Figure 1.1 Flowchart of the psychoanalytic consultation hour's process.

SECOND STEPS: two clinical examples

The survival strategy: fighting for women's rights (report M. Leuzinger-Bohleber)

When arriving in Germany in 2016, Mrs E. was in a state of shock, socially completely isolated, suffering from severe sleep and eating disorders. Her husband was at a loss, feared that she would take her own life. Mrs E. had fled Kurdistan, where she had worked hard for women's rights as a deputy mayor. The Turkish police had overrun her village one day, rounded up women and their children in one place, and brutally murdered them. Mrs E. herself had only narrowly escaped this situation. She could not forgive herself for not being able to save her three girlfriends, who called her by cell phone, desperate and badly wounded. When we talked about her unbearable feelings of survivor guilt, she started to cry violently. Her husband took her into his arms and looked at me helplessly. "Can you do something that she stops crying . . . ?" he said. "I think she has really deep reasons to cry, this is the language of the psyche. Crying is better than just being frozen . . ., " I answered. And indeed, in the second crisis intervention session, she was in a somewhat better state and consoled herself with the thought that she could continue to work for women's rights – also here in "Michaelisdorf." We supported her very much in this. In addition, she, a physicist with a doctorate, became involved in language courses, since she had already been to Germany as a teenager and therefore spoke German quite well.

She had therefore found a first way out of the acute traumatisation and developed an attitude that Jonathan Lear describes as *"radical hope":* Full of verve, she wanted to get involved with Kurdish women here in Germany, to become politically active together with her husband (e.g., by reporting on the brutal persecution by the Turkish Army in a Kurdish newspaper in exile) (Sperry & Mull, 2021).

After one and a half years she contacted me unexpectedly. She had broken down again and was in a terrible mental state. As we have often seen with refugees, after a *latency period* in which they feel relatively well and have used all their psychic energy to arrive in Germany, learn the language, take care of their asylum application, find a place to live, work, and so on, they are caught up again by the unsolved traumatic experience: They break down again and now seek therapeutic help in psychotherapies that go beyond crisis intervention and allow for a more in-depth processing of the traumatic experiences.

In Mrs E.'s case, it was the death of her father that had led to the breakdown. Flooded with horror and panic, she described holding him dying in her arms. Seeing the blood pouring from his nose and mouth, she was suddenly flooded with horrific images: as already mentioned, she had seen dying mothers and children bleeding to death, shot by Turkish soldiers in the public square outside her office in her small Kurdish town.

The images were part of embodied memories of these traumatic experiences (Leuzinger-Bohleber, 2018) and combined with olfactory and auditory hallucinations: the soldiers had set fire to houses where refugees were hiding; she heard their screams, smelt the burnt bodies – and heard, over and over again – the voices of her friends on her cell phone . . ..

In the now regular psychoanalytic therapy (beginning end of 2017), we understood that the death of her father had reactivated her unresolved oedipal conflicts. She had never detached herself from him as an oedipal figure. She had used massive idealisation to ward off her extreme anger and hatred of him. The father had massively libidinously seduced her, as his only daughter, on the one hand. He had enormously stimulated her oedipal desires for superiority over her mother, who was an uneducated woman from a farm in Kurdistan while he himself had an academic degree. On the other hand, he had repeatedly extremely devalued and humiliated his daughter by his patriarchal behaviour. Only very late did she dare to enter into a sexual relationship with a much older man and marry. However, unconsciously, she experienced her marital relationship as incestuous and therefore renounced having children. Her father had fled to Germany already in the 1990s. After having arrived in Germany as a refugee, she took care of him, who suffered from severe dementia, for over one year until his death. Mrs E. unconsciously experienced the images of the dying man as a confirmation of her own sadistic-destructive, murderous fantasies, which led to horrible feelings of guilt and a renewed breakdown.

Therefore, the psychoanalytic work in the following months revolved very much around the collapse of the idealisation of the paternal object and, connected with it, her female self-image as a "good, holy woman," which seemed close to a self-idealisation,[3] who always took the side of the "good," "right," and who dedicated her entire life to the commitment for more rights for women in her Muslim country, connected with a vision of a political liberation of her oppressed country. The traumatic experiences related to the brutal attack by the Turkish Army; the extreme helplessness and powerlessness of not being able to save her girlfriends; but also the failure of all her political activities as well as the subsequent flight, in which she was separated from her husband and sexually humiliated in a Turkish prison and only narrowly escaped rape had led to the outlined psychological breakdown, a psychic shock, and a severe dissociative state.

The psychoanalytic work in 2018 was very painful for her despite my professional holding and containing functions in which I tried to re-establish at least in parts a basic trust in good inner objects which had been destroyed during her traumatic experiences.[4] Obviously, this had a great influence on her: she regained some of her activity and creativity, and together with me, she dared to find images and words for the atrocities she had gone through. Writing them down obviously fulfilled a therapeutic function for her.

Through therapy, as Luci (2017, 2021) describes it, a kind of second skin seemed to form around Mrs E., carefully overlaying the traumatically destroyed one (Anzieu, 2014).

But then Mrs E. experienced another personal catastrophe: she suffered a severe stroke and only narrowly escaped death. She largely lost her speech and mobility, so she had to spend months in a rehabilitation clinic. It was no longer possible for her to continue therapy. From time to time, we tried to telephone, or she wrote me, with the help of her husband, an email – a very sad, tragic story, which confronted me painfully, and once again in a completely unexpected way, with the limits of what is psycho-analytically possible.

As I continue to be preoccupied with the psychoanalytic process that has begun with Mrs E. in connection with the attempt to enable her to regain some rudimentary access to her own destructive-aggressive impulses, and therefore also to her vitality and self-agency in combination with re-establishing some kind of a basic trust in a helping other, I would like to summarise an analogous therapeutic concern in another treatment that has been very much on my mind during the months of the pandemic. My guess is that the extreme traumatisation due to torture, war, and persecution for all refugees, women and men, have extreme psychic consequences, especially in coping with their own vital, aggressive impulses. As I would like to illustrate, this leads to a challenging therapeutic focus to enable these people to regain some sense of self-agency and connectedness with others.

The fight against inner persecution: from the psychotherapy with Mr A.

Like Mrs E., Mr A. had also received several crisis intervention sessions in May 2017 as part of the pilot project STEP-BY-STEP at the first-arrival centre "Michaelisdorf" in Darmstadt. He was severely suicidal and suffered from severe depression and panic attacks. He showed all symptoms of a posttraumatic stress disorder. The crisis intervention offered there was successful: the patient rejoined social life in "Michaelisdorf," worked in the carpentry workshop, and cared for other traumatised refugees. He completed a professional internship in a small handicraft business and proved to be a reliable, valued employee, so that the head of the company eventually offered him a permanent position. He completed the language courses. With the help of drug treatment, he was relatively stable thanks to the care of a very dedicated psychiatrist and some supportive talks with me.

In the fall of 2019, however, he turned to me again. An upcoming operation had triggered a serious crisis. It turned out that the patient, in an adolescent phase of rebellion, had placed a tattoo on his back that expressed a defamatory slogan against those in power. The prospect that nurses or doctors would discover this tattoo in connection with surgery had led to a reactivation of the trauma. The tattoo had been discovered by the intelligence service of the Muslim country in 2014. He was arrested, tortured, and raped. He managed to escape prison but could only save his life by fleeing. First in Greece and then in Hungary, he was detained in refugee camps under inhumane conditions. Again, he was a victim of severe physical and psychological violence, which haunts him in nightmares to this day. Every time he was threatened with deportation to Hungary because of the Schengen Agreement during the last four years; this triggered panic and anxiety in him.

Since the last two years, Mr A. is in a regular psychoanalytic psychotherapy with me. At the moment we often focus on his aggressive-destructive impulses, which frighten him very much and had even plunged him into a psychotic episode. In the following paragraphs are some clinical observations, which I would like to illustrate – for the sake of brevity – by means of some central dreams.[5]

Shortly after his operation he told me the following dream:

> *I dreamed about my sister's husband. The one who needs surgery. He is a professional runner. I like him very much. . . . In the dream he lost both his legs – maybe in the war – I carried him on my back, but I didn't even dare to tell him that he lost his legs.*[6]

We talked about the dream image. In contrast to the regime of terror in his homeland, he felt pity for his brother-in-law and literally loaded him on his shoulders, a heavy burden that weighs him down.

Then he remembered another dream in the same session:

> *I'm back in X., on a country road. My father and uncle are with me. Our car breaks down. I am supposed to fix it. We open the hood. My father rips out all the hoses. He tells me to fix this. I just ask him why he did this.*

His associations lead to a connection between his father, as an authority figure in his culture, and torture. His father was loving. He never beat him. But the torturers, as representatives of the "fatherland," tortured him severely. All this is mixed in the dream. His father becomes a sadistic figure, as in the first dream he told me in Michaelis-Village, when his father wanted to drag him down to the open grave and reproaches him for abandoning his mother and fleeing. Then we talked again about my intervention at that time, which helped him get out of his suicidality. I said in the crisis intervention in 2017, "I am sure that your mother, who obviously loves you very much, would rather have a living son in Germany than a dead son in X." His (oedipal and preoedipal) feelings of guilt could be somewhat alleviated by this interpretation at that time, but were, of course, still psychically present. The guilty feelings seemed now, according to his own interpretation, to endanger his autonomy ("his car"). Is it allowed that he really gets ahead here in Germany, becomes autonomous and a bit independent from his family?[7]

This theme was one focus of the therapy during the following months. In a session some months later, he told again an important dream:

> Dream: "I was tortured, and I am disabled. I, can no longer walk, am paralyzed, cannot speak. I try to move. I want to tell the people around me, I'm just pretending. . . . Finally, I manage to move my hands. I gain more and more strength. I can even bend an iron – even my legs I can move again – : Then I take a knife and hurt one of my torturers badly in the neck. The other I slit the entire belly and tear out his intestines – "

"How can I do such a thing?" he said frightened.

We talked about the fact that it is understandable that he is frightened, that he brutally attacks his opponents in his dream, but that such impulses are awakened when one is tortured and made a disabled person. In the dream he regains his strength and his hands and his ability to fight back. This allows him to overcome the paralysed, (disabled) state of complete powerlessness and helplessness he experienced during the torture and regain access to his vitality, his sense that he can fight back. Important for him was my explanation that the dream finds drastic images for this, and it is therapeutically very important that he can remember this dream at all and approaches the important psychological truth that he is not only a passive victim, as in the second dream, but can also actively defend and protect himself (and his mother).

This theme was like a red thread in the therapeutic sessions of the last year and also emerged in the transference. To close with a short example of a session of the last weeks of treatment:

> Mr. A. reacted intensively to irregularities in our treatment as the recent example of a session last week shows. I had to reschedule a session. He did not accept the alternative appointment, but waived an hour last week. When I wanted to address this in the next session, he interrupted me with a remarkably rough voice. He told me that he is not feeling well. He had severe nightmares all night, he said, and was frightened that he had become aggressive in his job. "(This) I do not (want) to be this way. . . . I have always been a friendly person."

We talked about exactly what happened. He yelled at a colleague when he said he would not come to work.

> You can't do this. . . . I yelled at him. But I am not his boss – I was very ashamed, I don't want to go to work anymore. . . . (after a pause): In the dreams last night I cut the throats of many people with a

knife. Two people were very tall. The knife was blunt. I could not kill them. . . . Then these two persons approached me with knives.[8] I woke up in panic.

We talked about the fact that it was understandable that these dreams scared him a lot, because they attacked his central self-image as well as his self-ideal that he is a peaceful person (he belongs to a religious minority that preaches peace on earth).

> Nevertheless, we have seen from many of your dreams as well as in our therapeutic relationship (when e.g., you dared to tell me how insulted you have been because I had to cancel a session last week) how important it is that, after your capability to actively resist injustice has broken down in torture, you regain your activity and not remain just the passive victim. . . . Only by doing so can you become healthy and protect yourself and your loved ones.

I reminded him of these dreams and his stories from childhood, how little it was allowed in his family and in his culture "to be aggressive," but that from an early age on, he was required "to be kind," "to be silent," and "not to hit, to hurt others physically," and so on.[9]

> Also, for this reason it is probably very difficult for your psyche to differentiate between the "healthy" need to resist injustice and to be active and the "murderous-brutal" impulses, which were both forbidden in your family, but also, moreover, mixed with the terrible traumatic experiences during the torture. In no case did you want to become like your torturers.

These interpretations seemed to reach him. We could talk about the fact that, moreover, as a tolerated refugee in Germany, it would be quite dangerous for him in real terms if he would get involved in aggressive conflicts. Therefore, he had the idea to talk to his boss about his current difficulty due to his psychotherapeutic "healing process," which was connected to his temporary difficulty to control his affects and to ask his boss for his understanding and tolerance.

It was amazing that working through the topic of his own aggressive-destructive impulses mainly in the transference relationship with me led to his courage to look for a romantic love partner on the internet. Three weeks after this session, he reported that he had a very nice date with a well-educated, differentiated woman of his age, a refugee from another country than himself. He was full of hope to finally find someone he could share his life with and thus would feel less lonely here in Germany.

Summary and discussion

With two short case studies we wanted to illustrate that it seems possible to work psychoanalytically in depth with refugees, but often only in the sense of a "SECOND STEP," when they – supported by "FIRST STEPS" in the initial-reception facilities – were able to arrive in the external reality in Germany. After such *a latency period*, it is often the reactivation of unresolved unconscious conflicts, which are linked to embodied memories of trauma, torture, persecution, and flight that motivates the refugees to seek longer-term psychoanalytic treatment.

At the same time, we hoped to illustrate how much the analyst is confronted with his personal and professional limitations in these treatments – for example, because he has to cope with the unbearable trauma in his countertransference and his recurring ambivalences in the confrontation with the foreign, which constantly make him realise how little he really knows and understands about the different countries of origin, cultures, educational practices, ideals, and value systems and so on of his refugee patient. Nevertheless, in contemporary psychoanalysis, there seems to exist a broad body of knowledge about psychic reactions of human beings *that seem to be ubiquitous to all individuals, women and men, who have suffered extreme trauma*, such as:

- The breakdown of self-agency and basic trust in a helping other.
- The regression to omnipotent thinking in order to defend against helplessness and a turn from passive to active by psychically assuming (counter to the facts) one's own responsibility for the traumatic event.
- A frozen sense of time as a consequence of the traumatisation as well as an unconsciously produced standstill of life time.
- The predominance of a self-object fusion as the core of traumatic experience.
- The deep anxiety to identify with the aggressor and the loss of a productive handling of one's own aggressive impulses.
- Nightmares and flashbacks as failed attempts to mentalise embodied memories of the suffered traumatisation, and so on.[10]

We could not address in the frame of this chapter the fact that (due to our experiences) it is important to first understand and treat these ubiquitous consequences of extreme traumatisation in psychoanalytic therapies as well as cultural and gender-specific conflicts and fantasies.

To conclude: In view of the worldwide migration of peoples, often connected with trauma, flight, and displacement, it seems to be the order of the day that we, as psychoanalysts, with our specific knowledge of the unconscious, engage in the care of traumatised refugees, women and men.

We try to give a language to their embodied memories of the unbearable, even if we can never really heal the wounds of extreme traumatisation.

Part II

Psychotherapeutic approach in a psychosocial centre for refugees (Gertraud Schlesinger-Kipp)

After the international conference of the IPA in Boston 2015, during which much was said on the challenges to psychoanalysis in this changing world, we Germans came back to another rapidly changing reality. Escaping the terror of the IS, not drowning in the Mediterranean like so many others, fleeing the tent cities in Lebanon, Jordan, Turkey by the millions, hiking around the Hungarian barbwire fences in the mud, they ended up with us (1.1 million in 2015, Germany). The causes for escaping and taking refuge in this world exist not only since this summer of 2015, but the misery hadn't been this clear and close for a long time.

Alexander and Margarete Mitscherlich were psychoanalysts who meddled in the present after World War II. The Psychoanalytical Institute in Kassel, with the name and in the tradition of Alexander-Mitscherlich-Institute (DPV/IPA) organised in 2015 until today 20–25 psychoanalysts, as well as psychiatrists and psychotherapists and child and adolescent analysts have come together to share their feelings and fears and thoughts, and to organise help for the refugees.

In the countries where the refugees come from, there are dehumanising states and experiences, not only in the war but also on the escape route and at our border fences and now in Germany as well. We believe that psychoanalysis and we, as persons, can approach the question and try to understand how these dehumanising processes affect the individual, now and in the long term. This means also not to dehumanise ourselves. Meanwhile, we know from trauma research that the manner how the refugees are welcomed or not is essential for further psychic and social development. We believe that we can contribute to inhibit radicalisation and criminalisation and foster integration. The big difference to the mass migration in many other countries of the world is here in Europe that there are different cultures, religions, and languages, so the integration process is crucial for the society. Because for them we are strangers, many have given up everything they owned. In Syria, for example, they had a completely normal family life in their culture, work, training, school, studies, and possessions. The refugees from Afghanistan, on the other hand, have known nothing but war for generations, which destroys family ties and makes society unsympathetic and cruel to weaker people and children. Often, families have fled back and forth between Iran and Afghanistan for years. On the other hand, for refugees, the encounter with someone who exposes himself or herself, like we therapists, to their foreignness, therefore, already creates a small piece of healing (Schlesinger-Kipp, 2019).

Most often, we found posttraumatic stress disorder (PTSD) in various manifestations. Many of the refugees lost relatives during the escape and/or have contact with family members who still are under life threat in their home countries. Almost as often, residents with depression, anxiety, and panic disorders were introduced to us, which sometimes existed already in the home country, and often it came to marital and family problems with much violence and drug abuse.

In 2015–2016 psychoanalytic groups in Hesse founded specific centres for supporting refugees (in Frankfurt, Gießen, Kassel), where refugees in psychic pain and hopeless situations find psychosocial counselling and psychotherapeutic help. In 2016 a group of psychoanalysts founded the Psychosocial Centre in Kassel, financed by the government in Hesse (Kramuschke et al., 2016).

After the number of new refugees declined, many first-arrival institutions have been closed. However, the three Psychosocial Centres in Hesse are still working, even in times of the coronavirus pandemic, which has proven to be particularly difficult for refugees. The most frequent problem at the moment is the impending deportation to the home country because asylum is not acknowledged (more than one-third of these decisions are not valid before the court and have to be withdrawn in favour of the refugees) or to the European country where they first entered. This is often Italy or Greece, and you can imagine what happens if the refugee has to go back there. These countries are left alone by the EU with their border problems and are struggling with the masses of refugees coming through the Mediterranean Sea.

Escape and gender

According to the council of German psychotherapists, about 40% of the refugees are mentally ill or traumatised (Sé Holovko & Schlesinger-Kipp, 2019).

One-third of all refugees, who in January 2016 for the first time applied for asylum in Germany, are women and girls. They leave their homeland necessarily for the same reasons as men: war, bombed cities, villages under ISIS rule, no water, no electricity, no food, no future, shattered lives, and political oppression. There are also gender-specific reasons for escape: domestic violence, forced marriages, female genital mutilation, honour killings. For women, the escape is – on foot, in unfit boats, in trains – usually more dangerous than for men. They are even more vulnerable to physical, sexual, and psychic violence than men. Even here in the refugee camps, many run the risk of suffering sexual violence by partners, residents, or even personnel. While the men try to be mobile, women almost never leave their accommodation out of fear and because it was not common in their countries of origin to walk alone in the street.

Gender-related persecution applies since 1951 (Geneva Convention) as reason for asylum, but this was recognised only since 2005 by the Immigration Act in Germany. In reality, last year, out of more than 33,000 applicants for asylum in Germany, only 624 were recognised because of "gender-related persecution in their home country," which are mainly women, but also homosexual men. Often proofs are required that the women cannot bring.

In all wars since ancient times, rape of women and other forms of sexual violence was and is used by the war combatants to destroy procreation, to serve the soldiers to be able to do the war work, to fuse ones genes into the enemy, to humiliate the enemy, to attack the most fragile part of the enemy (ie, women and girls). In many countries women are considered as less valuable, less worthy as individuals. Fatal outcomes of this are more homicides and suicides, more unintended pregnancies, miscarriages and stillbirth, preterm delivery, and low birth weight of babies. Depression in young mothers is common as well as posttraumatic stress and other disorders; sleep and eating disorders; psychosomatic problems such as headache, back pain, fibromyalgia; psychic and actual retreat; and poor overall health (S. Varvin).

Creating guidelines for therapeutic sessions (Kramuschke & Schlesinger-Kipp, 2016)

In the frame of the Psychosocial Centre Kassel, we usually can offer just a few therapeutic sessions. We have developed the following short guideline for psychoanalytic therapists:

1. Opening of the conversation:

- Building up trust
- Introduction by confidant (interpreter)
- Secrecy, volunteer work, no political authority

2. Trauma

- "What was the worst?" Individual traumatic story
- Respect the unspeakable
- Refugee should not be overwhelmed by painful emotions
- Sympathy, expressing compassion

3. Relieve feelings of shame and guilt

- Shame by identity and dignity loss
- Shame as a victim of violence
- De-pathologisation
- Guilt feelings as a survivor

4. End of the offer

- Do not leave in helpless situation
- Address resources and coping
- Discuss practical help

Short case study

An unaccompanied 17-year-old minor from an African country, Nouri, is announced in May 2020. She appears very shy, roundish in the face, with a hijab tight around her neck. The interpreter is missing. The centre worker finds a pregnant interpreter by phone, but it is not clear what is going on. However, as the caregiver at the facility makes it urgent that we speak to Nouri, another attempt is made. In the next conversation with an interpreter, Nouri tells us the following:

She lived in a village with her parents and three little brothers. In her country, men from a clan that "owns" the region seek out young women by simply taking them with them. There was a knock, and she opened the door with a little brother in her arms. A man grabbed her wrist hard and the brother fell down. Her father came and tried to help her. Then the men shot him and the little brother. Her mother then immediately sent her to a doctor and a friend, who immediately helped her escape via two different African countries to finally arrive in Libya. She lived there in a camp/prison for one year and experienced a lot of violence there. It is difficult for her to talk about it. They treated her "like an animal," she says. That is all we can find out in this session. The interpreter and I are very depressed by this story.

The next time, the interpreter is simply not there. I had the feeling that she could not bear the story.

The staff member gives me her mobile phone with a translation program, but it fails. I had the feeling that Nouri – because of the emotional strain of it all – cannot read at all. I get the idea that maybe she can't read her mother tongue at all and ask a staff member how I can respectfully find out. She says I could ask how it was at school at home when I get a chance.

July '20

In the next session, we have a new interpreter who is very sensitive but clear. We are with her until the end of the talks. We learn on occasion when asked that Nouri has never attended school. When we came to talk about her difficulties at school here, I asked her what it was like at school, at home, and it came out. She had never mentioned this to her teachers here. Her mother had taught her to read and write a little.

I would have had a hard time with these conversations without this new interpreter. The interpreter translates in a motherly mood. It is obviously good for the patient to hear her own language. We ask a lot about her life before she fled, on the farm with her brothers and parents, to bring her home a bit closer. I keep telling her that the girl inside her is broken but is still there, that she will find the girl inside again. I ask the interpreter if they understand (because I don't know if this professional speak is understandable), and they both nod vigorously. She tells me how nice it was as the eldest with her mother in the field and how they played with the little brothers. Therefore, she has a good inner object on which to base the processing of her traumatisation.

In the next session, she seems happier. She has found her mother! An aunt and other women from her home country have helped her, and tomorrow there will be a phone call with the mother. She is happy and excited.

October '20

After the summer holidays, Nouri is very withdrawn and depressed. Yes, she spoke to her mother on the phone. She and the brothers are fine. Nouri only talks about longing for her mother. She needs her mother. She wants to bring them to Germany; this is sometimes possible for unaccompanied minors. The Youth Welfare Office wants to help her, but she has to find €500. How is she supposed to do that?

She cannot sit next to boys at school. She talks in more detail about her experiences in prison and camps in Libya. I will spare you that here. I repeat several times that it is not hers to feel shame but should be the perpetrators shame.

November '20

She looks different. She says that she has already collected €400 for her mother, 200 from her aunt, and 200 she collected at school.

She spoke in class and collected these €200 there! We confirm to her how brave she is now to speak in class (also about the lack of schooling). I look for (and find) a place for her at a child's therapist. However, the counsellor at the facility says that she does not want that now. The talks with me had helped her a lot, but she did not want to talk about it anymore. In the meantime, however, she has arrived at the therapist.

Working with the interpreter was very helpful here. If only to be able to contain the traumatic life of Nouri and thus also to give her some self-confidence. Also, the pressure to act, which is often great for us and especially for the interpreters (like ours – of course, reflected and repressed – wish for immediate help (eg, pulling €100 out of our own pockets)), can be shared in the follow-up discussion. To regain self-agency for the refugee, it is sometimes important to restrain from too much helping.

Notes

1 Marianne Leuzinger-Bohleber and Nora Hettich have been in responsible positions for FIRST STEPS in the "Michaelisdorf." The scientific evaluation of STEP-BY-STEP was part of the political legitimation to establish by 2017 three Psychosocial Centres in Hesse, in North Hesse (Kassel/Giessen), one in middle Hesse (Frankfurt), and one in the South of Hesse (Darmstadt). Gertraud Schlesinger-Kipp is one of the founders of the Psychosocial Centre in Kassel, which offers psychotherapeutic and psychosocial support in the first-reception camp and after they have left the initial-reception centres.

2 A screening carried out by various groups working in the "Michaelisdorf" had proven to be very successful. On the other hand, we have dropped the use of "objective questionnaires" (self-assessments) because it had been shown that the refugees often ticked off the "desired answers" (for example, they hinted at severe trauma when they suspected that this increases their chance to stay in Germany). In a pilot study (supported by the IDeA Center, Center for Adaptive and Individual Development and Adaptive Education for Children-at-Risk), 60 refugees were assessed with a semi-standardised interview (modified approach of the Socio-Economic Panel (SOEP)). These interviews were very fruitful in terms of scientific gain as well as in terms of preventive options.

3 Self-idealisation seemed to be a necessary defence mechanism of many severely traumatised refugees in order to survive the humiliation, degradation, and even dehumanisation of trauma.

4 Another central aspect of the therapeutic work was that we successively understood better how much she was fused with the killed objects and literally carried "dead objects" within her in her inner object world (as Freud had already described in *Mourning and Melancholia* (Freud, 1914)). Moreover, it became apparent that she had also unconsciously identified with the perpetrator, a reason why she remained in a state of shock, an extreme passivity in the sense of a kind of "dead reflex." Unconsciously, every activity was equated with the actions of the torturers. To do nothing was therefore an unconscious attempt not to identify with the aggressor.

5 It is astonishing that Mr A. – in contrast to many traumatised refugees – could remember the contents of his nightmares, an indication that he had not completely lost his ability to mentalise due to the extreme traumatisation.

6 The manifest dream content hints to the fusing of his inner objects; the injured man seems also be part of his own body image.

7 His abysmal loneliness – brought about by his massive conflict of loyalties; his feelings of survivor's guilt; but also his individual, familial, and cultural uprooting – was psychologically alleviated unconsciously, among other things, by the fact that he remained very much identified with his primary objects. Thus, in a session in which he dreamed that his mother was visiting him in his apartment here in Germany, we found the formulation: "It is enough if 50% of your soul is in X., with your family but 50% here in Germany. Your mother allows you in the dream to feel comfortable here in your apartment, in Germany." This theme was also connected to his feeling that his lifetime had been frozen: a basic feeling of continuity of past, present, and future had broken down during the experiences of extreme trauma (Cournut, 1988).

8 This is another indicator for the fusion of his inner objects: he is victim and perpetrator at the same time and struggles to separate his inner objects, his self and object representations. These processes have also been connected by negative fantasies of omnipotence as a defence of the experience of extreme helplessness during trauma.

9 I cannot go into the topic of the cultural and gender-specific socialisation of boys in the Muslim countries where castration anxieties seem to be stimulated very much by the abrupt separation of the boys from their mother as well as by the late circumcision (when the boys are between five and six years) (Akhtar, 2010; Appadurai, 2013; Karakaşoğlu, 2015; Khoshrouy-Sefat, 2007; Kristeva, 1990).

10 In addition, it should be mentioned at least briefly, that in the meantime, broad psychoanalytical and interdisciplinary knowledge have been collected on (ubiquitous and specific) reactions to flight and migration in general (loss of family, home, group identities, the protective skin of culture, of togetherness and shared values and ideals, etc.; uprooting of the self, guilt feelings and loyalty conflicts in context with leaving behind the beloved ones, survivor's guilt and self-punishment, failed mourning processes, etc.) (e.g., special issues of *Journal of Applied Psychoanalytic Study*, 2019, edited by Leuzinger-Bohleber & Parens, 2018, and of *Psychoanalytic Inquiry*, February/March 2021, edited by Lichtenberg & Bronstein and references).

References

Akhtar, S. (2010). *Immigration and acculturation: Mourning, adaptation, and the next generation*. Maryland: Jason Aronson.

Anzieu, D. (2014). *The group and the unconscious (RLE: Group therapy)*. London: Routledge.

Appadurai, A. (2013). The future as cultural fact: Essays on the global condition. *Rassegna Italiana Di Sociologia, 14*(4), 649–650.

Bohleber W. (2010). *Destructiveness, intersubjectivity and trauma: The identity crisis of modern psychoanalysis*. London: Karnac Books.

Cournut, J. (1988). Ein Rest, der verbindet. Das unbewußte Schuldgefühl, das Entlehnte betreffend. *Jahrbuch Der Psychoanalyse, 22*, 67–98.

Erikson, E. H. (1959). *Identity and the life cycle: Selected papers*. Madison: International Universities Press.

Fonagy, P., Luyten, P., Allison, E., & Campbell, C. (2019). Mentalizing, epistemic trust and the phenomenology of psychotherapy. *Psychopathology, 52*(2), 94–103. https://doi.org/10.1159/000501526

Freud, S. (1914). Mourning and melancholia, the standard edition of the complete psychological works of Sigmund Freud, ed. James Strachey et al. *Hogarth Press, 1916*(14), 239–260.

Geiselberger, H. (2017). *Die große Regression: Eine internationale Debatte über die geistige Situation der Zeit*. Berlin: Suhrkamp Verlag.

Hettich, N. (in review). *Fragile hope – A grounded theory on psychosocial support for accompanied adolescent refugees in German reception centers*.

Hettich, N., & Meurs, P. (2021). Complex dynamics in psychosocial work with unaccompanied minor refugees with uncertain future prospects: A case study. *International Journal of Applied Psychoanalytic Studies, 18*(1), 41–57. https://doi.org/10.1002/aps.1676

Hettich, N., Seidel, F. A., & Stuhrmann, L. Y. (2020). Psychosocial Interventions for newly arrived adolescent refugees: A systematic review. *Adolescent Research Review, 5*(2), 99–114. https://doi.org/10.1007/s40894-020-00134-1

Karakaşoğlu, Y. (2015). Islam und Moderne, Bildung und Integration. Einstellungen türkisch-muslimischer Studentinnen erziehungswissenschaftlicher Fächer. In M. Rumpf, U. Gerhard, & M. M. Jansen (Eds.), *Facetten islamischer Welten* (pp. 272–289). Transcript Verlag. Retrieved from www.degruyter.com/document/doi/10.14361/9783839401538-013/html.

Khoshrouy-Sefat, H. (2007). Migration und seelische Krankheit: Analytische Psychotherapie mit Migranten aus traditionsgeleiteten Gesellschaften – speziell aus dem Iran. *Zeitschrift für Individualpsychologie, 32*(3), 245–264. https://doi.org/10.13109/zind.2007.32.3.245

Kramuschke, P., & Schlesinger-Kipp, G. (2016). Möglichkeiten und Grenzen einmaliger therapeutischer Gespräche mit Geflüchteten in Erstaufnahmeeinrichtungen. In *DPV Tagungsband*. Gießen: Psychosozial Verlag.

Kramuschke, P., Schlesinger-Kipp, G., & Kreusch, U. (2016). Flüchtlinge: Verborgenes Leid ist doppeltes leid. *Hessisches Ärzteblatt, 6*, 336–339.

Kristeva, J. (1990). *Fremde sind wir uns selbst*. Frankfurt, New York: Edition Suhrkamp.

Latour, B. (2017). *Facing Gaia: Eight lectures on the new climatic regime*. New Jersey: John Wiley & Sons.

Leuzinger-Bohleber, M. (2015). Working with severely traumatized, chronically depressed analysands. *The International Journal of Psychoanalysis, 96*(3), 611–636. https://doi.org/10.1111/1745-8315.12238

Leuzinger-Bohleber, M. (2016). From free speech to IS – Pathological regression of some traumatized adolescents from a migrant background in Germany. *International Journal of Applied Psychoanalytic Studies, 13*(3), 213–223. https://doi.org/10.1002/aps.1499

Leuzinger-Bohleber, M. (2018). *Finding the body in the mind: Embodied memories, trauma, and depression*. London: Routledge.

Leuzinger-Bohleber, M., & Hettich, N. (2018). *"Fremd bin ich eingezogen . . . " STEP-BY-STEP: Ein Pilotprojekt zur Unterstützung von Geflüchteten in einer Erstaufnahmeeinrichung*. Berlin: Psychosozial Verlag.

Leuzinger-Bohleber, M., Rickmeyer, C., Tahiri, M., Hettich, N., & Fischmann, T. (2016). What can psychoanalysis contribute to the current refugee crisis? *The International Journal of Psychoanalysis, 97*(4), 1077–1093.

Leuzinger-Bohleber, M., Tahiri, M., & Hettich, N. (2017). STEP-BY-STEP: Pilotprojekt zur Unterstützung von Geflüchteten in der Erstaufnahmeeinrichtung "Michaelisdorf" in Darmstadt. *Psychotherapeut, 62*(4), 341–347. https://doi.org/10.1007/s00278-017-0208-6

Löwenthal, L. (1990). *Untergang der Dämonologien: Studien über Judentum, Antisemitismus und faschistischen Geist*. Berlin: Reclam-Verlag.

Luci, M. (2017). Disintegration of the self and the regeneration of 'psychic skin' in the treatment of traumatized refugees. *Journal of Analytical Psychology, 62*(2), 227–246. https://doi.org/10.1111/1468-5922.12304

Luci, M. (2021). The psychic skin between individual and collective states of mind in trauma. *Journal of Psychosocial Studies, 14*(1), 33–45.

Nachtwey, O. (2017). Entzivilisierung. Über regressive Tendenzen in westlichen Gesellschaften. In H. Gesielberger (Ed.), *Die grosse Regression. Eine internationale Debatte über die geistige Situation der Zeit* (pp. 215–231). Berlin: Suhrkamp.

Parens, H. (2014). *War is not inevitable: On the psychology of war and aggression.* Washington DC: Lexington Books.

Schlesinger-Kipp, G. (2019). Das Unheimliche in der Arbeit mit Geflüchteten. In *DPV Tagungsband* (pp. 210–214). Berlin: Psychosozial Verlag.

Sé Holovko, C., & Schlesinger-Kipp, G. (2019). Speaking of sexual abuse with female refugees. In P. Montagna & A. Harris (Eds.), *Psychoanalysis, law, and society.* London: Routledge.

Sperry, M., & Mull, S. (2021). Life on the line: Border stories. *Psychoanalytic Inquiry,* 41(2), 115–127.

Volkan, V. D. (2018). *Immigrants and refugees: Trauma, perennial mourning, prejudice, and border psychology.* London: Routledge.

2 A quite "normal" treatment with a refugee in the form of the International Clinic as part of the training outpatient clinic at the Frankfurt Psychoanalytic Institute

Annabelle Starck, Željko Čunović and Rosalba Maccarrone Erhardt

Part I

In Frankfurt, the tradition of psychoanalysis dates back to the 1920s. Its history contains forced emigration, displacement, persecution, and return. In 1926, the southwest German workgroup was created. In 1929 the first Frankfurt Psychoanalytic Institute (FPI) was founded with the support of the Institute of Social Science and Max Horkheimer.

Managed by Karl Landauer and Heinrich Meng, among the first colleagues were Frida Fromm-Reichmann, Erich Fromm, and Siegmund Heinrich Fuchs (later known in London as S. H. Foulkes). After the National Socialists seizure of power, the FPI was closed in 1933, and the involved analysts were forced into emigration. Karl Landauer died in the Bergen-Belsen concentration camp in 1945.

In 1960, with the support of Max Horkheimer, a new "Institute and Training Clinic for Psychoanalysis and Psychosomatic Medicine" was founded. The institute was managed by Alexander Mitscherlich and in 1964 renamed the "Sigmund-Freud-Institute" (SFI). In 1995, with the sole focus of the SFI on psychoanalytic research and its applications in cooperation with the universities of Frankfurt and Kassel, today's FPI (Frankfurt Psychoanalytic Institute) was founded (see Plänkers et al., 1996).

With the assumption of the former name of the institute, the new FPI wanted to continue in the traditions of the originally founded Frankfurt Psychoanalytic Institute as well as keeping the remembrance of the persecution alive. Today at the FPI, physicians and psychologists gain psychoanalytic training based on the statutes of the DPV and IPA. Integrated into

DOI: 10.4324/9781003203223-4

that is a training in psychodynamic psychotherapy[1] (in Germany, this is referred to as depth-based psychotherapy).

The outpatient department of the institute developed greatly over the years. The indication of psychoanalytic treatment broadened considerably. Today, not only is the "classical neurosis" considered treatable by psychoanalytic therapy, but the whole diverse spectrum of psychological suffering is treated in the outpatient clinic.

The treatment of people with negative migration experiences was specifically included in the treatment at the FPI. Difficulty in processing experiences and the suffering from the aftermath of escape and trauma after persecution developed into a focal point.

Migration and the treatment of migrants became the focus of many Frankfurt colleagues over the years. In the '80s and '90s, several projects emerged, putting the focus on the psychological implications of voluntary and forced migration. In the '90s publications about this topic intrigued several candidates and members of the FPI, leading to the founding of the "International Clinic" as a workgroup in the outpatient department. The group focuses on questions about the characteristics of the treatment in the native language of the patient as well as the connotations of analytic interactions between individuals from different cultures, especially the transference-countertransference relationship (Scheifele, 2021).

At that time, some of us already treated victims of political persecution and severe trauma. Despite the grievous personal history of many psychoanalysts, this practice was looked at with scepticism. It was seen as difficult to find an indication or an angle of psychoanalytical approach with uprooted and traumatised patients.

In 1993, the FATRA association (Frankfurt Workgroup Trauma & Exile) (Čunović, 2018) was founded in Frankfurt. This psychoanalytically orientated interdisciplinary institution offered consulting hours in a housing complex for refugees and developed into a treatment centre for refugees and tortured individuals using a psychoanalytical approach.[2]

In 2003 the first "Psychotherapy-Network for Refugees" was founded by FATRA in close cooperation with the FPI and SFI. It was joined by all psychoanalytic institutions in Frankfurt. In that way, reservations about psychoanalytical treatment for patients with issues caused by emigration, persecution, and trauma were eased into the therapeutic community. All interested analysts could participate in the network. If they treated traumatised refugees, they received support through supervision/collegial intervision and through regular specific professional lectures.

With the large wave of refugees reaching Europe and therefore Germany in 2015, an atmosphere of accommodation and willingness emerged. This "Culture of Welcome," which did not exist previously, developed.

The SFI engaged with several projects in research about the mental and psychological consequences of migration and escape led by Prof. Marianne Leuzinger-Bohleber since the beginning (see Leuzinger-Bohleber et al., 2016; Leuzinger-Bohleber & Hettich, 2018 or other contributions in this publication).

In 2015 the International Clinic was reactivated as an integrated part of the training institute offering help to refugees and migrants from Frankfurt and surroundings. Treatment could be sought independent of social or legal status, insurance, and irrespective of their knowledge of German. FPI members were engaged in the psychotherapy network for refugees for years and since 2015 were even more involved. For the first time, it was not just seen as possible but perceived as necessary that trainees were not just involved but trained to work with refugees. Since this work follows a genuine psychoanalytic approach, it is necessary to anchor these foundations in psychoanalytic training. The intensive exchange between seasoned colleagues and trainees was perceived as mutually beneficial. The direct questions from younger trainees and the often braver approaches to new challenges in treatment required of the experienced colleagues resulted in a constant reflection of their own practices and experiences. The exchange was facilitated in treatment seminars, free-of-charge supervisions and many lively clinical conferences. The IC (International Clinic) received hereby a new concept and could continue its work as part of the outpatient department (Čunović, 2019; Sturm, 2018).

Additionally, in 2017, the IC became part of the union "Psychosocial Association Rhein Main, Help for Refugees" (PSV), which comprises the Psychotherapy-Network for Refugees of 2003 and five organisations,[3] which are funded by the state of Hesse and offer psychosocial help to refugees. Here again, a regular interdisciplinary exchange is promoted by lectures, symposia, and seminars.

At present, with the Coronavirus pandemic, the number of colleagues engaged in the IC is slightly lower, and the excitement and enthusiasm diminished under the sorrows and worries caused by the pandemic.

Due to the pandemic, the placement of patients with colleagues for further treatment is possible only with greater engagement. Treatment opportunities for refugees are less than in the past. A positive situation exists, with several trainees completing part of their practical hours in an outpatient department and working in the IC. For some it seems that this opportunity is one of the reasons why they decide to train with the FPI.

When refugees are able to communicate sufficiently in German, their treatment is no different than the "usual" treatment. Nonetheless, the need for translation is sometimes still necessary. Working with three people in the therapeutic session is a special challenge and needs a lot of engagement by the trainee and the supervisor. Annabelle Starck will discuss this challenge in her case report.

Part II

Annabelle Starck

At the beginning of the initial interview, I encountered my 50-year-old patient, Ms A., huddled on a chair in the waiting area, covered with several scarves. She seemed old, small, and fragile. During my talk with this woman from Maghreb, I started to perceive her as much younger. I associated her with a baby bird that had fallen out of its nest. Motherly feelings spread through me creating an urge to care for this woman. I thought during our talk I could see a glimmer of hope in her eyes. She started to carefully and slowly talk about unconnected sequences of her life, offering information about her person.

I understood that she came to Germany with her son and daughter, as well as her granddaughter. She left her country of origin because of the political situation and to receive better medical care. Her daughter takes care of her and brought her here to our meeting.

In the following sessions, she sadly described that she could not go anywhere without help. She would experience strong fears, become disoriented, and forget where she was. She had difficulty sleeping. Closing her eyes would bring horrible visions, and when asleep, she described being haunted by nightmares. Additionally, throughout the day, she would slip into moments of overwhelming fear. She reports that she is also experiencing guilt and desperation over her need for her daughter's care. These feelings of guilt are understood as part of her depressive, self-accusing, but also omnipotent processing of traumatic experiences, as if she could have stopped past events from happening. These feelings of guilt are re-experienced in present relationships (eg, towards her daughter, in the transference).

She reports fragments of her experience of imprisonment with severe abuse and repeated sexualized violence. This was followed by hospitalisations and inadequate treatments, worsening her physical condition. I was overwhelmed, incredulous, and shaken by what this woman had to endure. I saw the tears flowing over her face and was terrified by the fear which I perceived.

When she started to talk more about her family background and her career path to a higher professional position, I started seeing her strong side. Her will to find safety in Germany was as remarkable as her wish to stay in touch with me. The change in her voice led me to see and imagine a less fragile "pre-traumatised" personality beginning to emerge.

A treatment by a trainee?

With the patient opening up, I felt that an analytical therapy could help her. Ms A. was hopeful to change her "burden" brought on by her feelings of guilt and her fear caused by intruding pictures. In the beginning I tried in vain to find somebody with the capacity to treat her. She always came back to me. In the meantime, I started treating patients and the question arose of "taking her with me" and treating her myself.

Since I am currently in training, the treatment situation has inherently special terms. It is a time of learning and insecurities, of dependence on assessments by supervisors. Sometimes it is similar to an ongoing exam situation. However, it is also a time of a secure frame, having my own ongoing training analysis and close, helpful supervision.

I thought about the always available Outpatient Clinic manager, the individual supervision, the Outpatient Clinic conference, the group supervision of the IC, my intervision group (where I always get important insights from my peers), and my training analysis. Čunović and Vukmanic (2000) emphasise the necessity of support by colleagues during the treatment of refugees, which was fulfilled in my case. Despite initial fears, a feeling of support and security emerged.

As usual, before a trainee treatment, an experienced colleague examined the case. She was concerned about a trainee taking over such a complex case. I was quite pleased when I received her final approval. It was as if Ms A. and I had passed a test.

Superficially argued by the premise that I did not have a third chair in my own practice, I began treatment sessions at the FPI. There are several floors with many rooms, colleagues, and constantly staffed Outpatient Department administration. Obviously, you are not alone but part of a whole. Also, for my patient, this perception was surely important. I observed during the month that she liked to come early before sessions and also liked to stay afterwards in the waiting area.

The involvement of an interpreter was necessary for my patient to express herself. She could use simple phrases in German but nothing more. Thanks to a pool of donations of the IC, which is supported by the members of the FPI, I could carry out my treatment with the support of an interpreter.[4]

At the onset of the therapeutic process, it became apparent that it was not solely the lack of a common language that caused confusion. Descriptions of experiences became blurred; times and dates were confused. Ms A. displayed dissociative states in varying degrees during our sessions. Regardless of my conviction that the opportunity for introspection was offered, the patient needed to avoid it to protect herself. I respected this defence mechanism, acknowledged it, and reflected on it with my supervisor. We deliberated that initially I would make myself available as an object to see which psychoanalytic processes would emerge.

Even though I was maintaining an absence of partisanship in our sessions, it was inevitable that we were getting closer to the traumatic experiences as well as her primary emotional relationships. It was apparent that one of our goals would be to achieve a narrative of her story to make a difference in processing possible.

A trainee treatment as a triad

I have dealt with the analytical therapeutic relationship. Now the question arose, what happens with this relationship when a third person is present?

With the inclusion of an interpreter, a third aspect is infused into the therapeutical dyad. This leads to the necessity of changing the basic conditions of the treatment (Čunović, 2019). The setting is changed.

We attempted to diminish the possible disturbance and influence of the interpreter on the therapeutic process. To achieve that, the role of the interpreter was defined and reflected in preliminary discussions and debriefings with the interpreter as well as in the supervision and during the sessions with the patient (Kluge & Kassim, 2006; Čunović, 2019). The interpreter contributes to the setting, which helps the patient and the therapist to maintain a frame and sometimes also orientation in rough terrain.

During supervisions this was frequently reflected. I was encouraged to talk to the interpreter afterwards to ask about her impressions.

In the beginning, the treatment was shaped by building a trusting relationship. Quickly a positive transference emerged. Nevertheless, in the beginning, the patient was hesitant to burden me and talk about difficult experiences.

Despite the positive aspects of an interpreter, it cannot be ignored that there is a controlling third entity in the room. The literary suggests that the therapist could feel less free (Miller et al., 2005). Nevertheless, the interpreter takes on triangulating features in this setting. Especially a highly traumatised patient who is threatened by regression might show tendencies to symbiotic processes in a tight analytic relationship. This can be relieved by the possibility of falling back on to a culturally close third person. Later in the treatment process I realised how the presence of the interpreter and the necessity of a translation protected me from being flooded by traumatic materials.

I am dependent on the translation; I am not able to talk to the patient on my own. There is no direct link through the meaning of the words. What is left is inflection and intonation which I can perceive as well as using the time spent translating to contemplate the dialogue.

The complexity of this relationship is also shown in the transference and countertransference. The perception and the differentiation of the transference and countertransference phenomena are difficult (Kluge & Kassim, 2006) and are, for me, ongoing challenges. Possibly my special situation as trainee (Baker et al., 2015) in frequent supervision plays a part here too.

Within the treatment process, on several occasions, the patient described a family-like feeling when she came to sessions. She perceived me and the interpreter as a unit. Simultaneously, in supervision, I understood that a special kind of daughter transference could be happening. Ms A. could have a positive (transference-) relationship with the interpreter and me as two additional daughters. She had a positive relationship with her children characterised by thankfulness, which was also relieved by our involvement.

At the same time, the patient also perceived herself as a child, in line with a regressive position towards me (Mother, Analyst), who repeatedly needed to assume auxiliary-ego-functions. This corresponds to her mother-daughter relationship. Likewise, her daughter is very supportive towards her, which was facilitated for both women by careful interpretation in the transference.

The mother-daughter relationship and the aspect of caring are recurring themes. Ms A. soon offers how her own mother was a strong and caring woman who always took an interest in others. However, her mother died early. In identification with her mother, she perceived herself in a similar light until her violent experiences occurred. The childlike-depending position, which she perceives towards her daughter and towards myself is exacerbating her feelings of guilt.

The trust in the treatment and the understanding of some biographic circumstances helped to strengthen her feeling of self rather quickly. With that, she started acting independently again. It moved me, when between appointments, she practiced her travel to the FPI with a friend, so she could make her way here independently.

Conflicting priorities between responsibility and not-knowing

In this treatment you can find two triangular constellations. On the one hand between patient, interpreter, and me as therapist. In this triangle everybody is situated in an "interspace" in which new aspects of understanding are emerging (Wohlfart et al., 2005). This journey is marked by resistances und misunderstandings. Despite the triangular setting, it was possible for me and the patient to form a relationship. I recall an interaction between me and the patient walking up the steps and her asking me with German intonation "And, good? Family good? All good?" She tried to initiate a direct contact with me. I answered her directly and thanked her while also smiling. With that a glow emerged on her face, which was strained from the exhaustion of walking up the steps. Later it was possible to discuss this scene in our treatment triangle. It became apparent that she wanted me to see her as a normal woman. With that, she was able to show the deep narcissistic wound caused by the abuse and the loss of her home and social status.

Possibly, before our treatment, the physical and mental weaknesses didn't leave space to grieve. She was fighting to survive and processed the experiences in a depressive-guilty fashion. It is apparent that her grown, independent part of the self, with functioning self-agency (see Bohleber, 2018) was lost repeatedly.

Over the course of our sessions, Ms A. started to perceive herself more and more in a grown-up position with a higher ego strength. She started making decisions increasingly on her own. When a possible change in her living situation caused much fear, she was able to voice her desire to stay in her living arrangement during the sessions. A letter written by me led to her being able to stay where she was. It was a long, fearful process, but the patient could decide her own situation by herself.

With that, I realised that I was feeling more secure, leading me to be able to form my own thoughts about important decisions in the course of the treatment. I perceived myself as increasingly independent. In doing so, the second triangle between me, the supervisor, and the patient helped me. During supervision I share everything that I perceive between me and the patient, me and the interpreter, and the patient and the interpreter. In this setting I have the possibility to reflect in the presence of a sympathetic third person.

I experienced myself in both triangles mostly as the "least knowing." The patient knows more about herself, the interpreter knows more about the country of origin, and the supervisor knows more about the technicalities of treatment. At the same time, I was the one to secure, intervene, and treat. This was often exhausting.

Surely my experiences were identified with Ms A., who needed to endure powerless, "not-knowing" in a foreign country but needed to act frequently. During the treatment process I started to realise that maybe it was more about enduring my "not-knowing" and reflecting on these feelings than to compensate for my "not-knowing" with knowledge.

Throughout supervisions I perceived increasingly that during interactions with the patient, the focus was on a joint discovery of her primary personality, of the central conflicts and the diverse processing connections with the traumatic experiences. On the one hand, I experience the cultural origin of Ms A. as well as her threatening violent experiences as an unknown and frightening terrain. On the other hand, I slowly started to feel, that in situations like these, it is necessary to acknowledge the lack of knowledge and work with what emerges in the present. Čunović describes this as a negative capability in the sense of Bion (*negative capability*, Bion, 1970), to bear the uncertainty, doubts, and inconsistencies, without trying to create facts (Čunović, 2019). Also, here the role as a trainee plays its part. I sometimes question myself if it is maybe more beneficial to bear insecurities, when you are feeling secure in your analytical stance.

Necessary interventions in the reality of the patient lead to further insecurities. As trainee I am constantly confronted with the difficulty of analytical abstinence. During the course of treatment, I found myself repeatedly in the situation of taking over auxiliary-ego-functions for the patient. The frame of the supervision supported me to not act blindly but to reflect on my doing and re-establish the broken abstinence. In hindsight, my insight into the necessity of concrete auxiliary-ego-actions possibly led to the patient's feeling of security and protection in our sessions and, hence, were supportive of her development. Regardless, interventions like that seem to me more justified if they are necessary and sufficiently reflected in their meaning (Čunović, 2019). After about one year, with her housing arrangement secured, the patient started talking about her imprisonment and rape. Piece by piece, she could remember fragments of her persecution experience. She feared that she might be responsible for the things that happened to her. This was exacerbated by her fear that indirectly she might be responsible for the death of a loved one. This topic was long avoided but, since coming to light, is central in the understanding of her situation by everybody involved.

In my opinion, it was important to refrain from urging or prompting her to talk about onerous material. It was crucial to give her the time and space to arrive at that point by herself – to feel the need to talk about it and experience the ego strength to do so. Over a long period of time, I worked containing, receiving, carefully clarifying, and interpreting without confrontation. The transference/countertransference relationship between us, especially in the manifold non-verbal aspects, was part of the reflection process since the beginning. Many fragments of her traumatic past were introduced into the analytical process at a later point. In part, by the patient, and in part, by myself, there are several steps apparent to moving from not knowing to knowing, from denying to narrating and understanding. Moving from a degree of remembering to a successive integration, which I understand like Laub and Auerhahn (1993) in the sense of a slow development of knowledge and experience continuum.

This was also possible during the Coronavirus pandemic. The patient's experiences with our triad continued during the lockdown, even when the sessions happened remotely. With the end of summer 2020, and our sessions continuing again in person, Ms A. started to introduce more and more dreams into our setting. It was possible to gain more understanding from them and put more and more pieces into a contextual and timely logical relation. We worked through the necessary differentiation between real risk of death and a resurgence of traumatic fears towards a recovery of her ability to experience a more reasonable worry.

Conclusion

The treatment is ongoing with almost 70 sessions over the course of two years (summer 2021). In the beginning, the sessions took place in a biweekly fashion, since the patient was considerably weak and involved in medical treatments. After transitioning into a weekly frequency of sessions, it was apparent that the sessions strengthened her instead of putting an additional burden on her. We are successful in slowly changing her traumatic reactions from feeling helpless to stronger self-agency and ego abilities in several new situations.

Overall, in this frame of a trainee-led treatment, it was successful in developing a secure relationship with the patient and to start an analytical developmental process. To that end, both triangles contributed. Much of my account shows the inner and outer workings of the patient, some of which may be influenced by the special setting and my trainee situation. Additionally, the unknown pandemic conditions contributed. It might be that the special frame with the interpreter, with a trainee as analyst, and frequent supervision (at least one hour supervision per four hours treatment) may have helped the collective endurance of the diverse insecurities and the "not-knowing" in this treatment of a refugee.

The encounter with Ms A. and other refugee patients personally brought me a special fulfilment and enrichment. To be trained in my apprenticeship to treat patients in such extraordinary and precarious situations is a necessity. In my opinion, this is vitally important for the development of contemporary psychoanalysis as well as for its social acceptability.

The patient herself described our treatment with the words "[Y]ou are trying with me to discover the roots and to care for them. A tree cannot be standing if you just care for the leaves."

Notes

1 This training can also be completed separately.
2 The former treatment centre is working today as a counselling centre for refugees from around the world.
3 FPI, SFI, FATRA, ERV (Evang. Regionalverband FF/M) and the Anna-Freud-Institute Frankfurt (AFI).
4 Despite the patient having regular health insurance and, subsequently, the right to stay in Germany, the insurance just pays for the treatment, but not for the interpreter.

References

Baker, S. W., Izzo, P., & Trenton, A. (2015). Psychodynamic considerations in psychotherapy using interpreters: Perspectives from psychiatry residents. *Psychodynamic Psychiatry*, 43(1), 117–128. doi:10.1521/pdps.2015.43.1.117.

Bion, W. R. (1970). *Attention and interpretation*. London: Tavistock Publications.

Bohleber, W. (2018, September 8). *Vortrag Neue Wege in der Behandlung traumatisierter Patienten*. Clinical Forum Series: Trauma – Praxis und Konzepte. Frankfurt: Frankfurt Psychoanalytik Institute.

Čunović, Ž. (2018). Anmerkungen zur Geschichte des Frankfurter Arbeitskreises Trauma und Exil, *fatra e.V.* Unpublished lecture manuscript.

Čunović, Ž. (2019). Analytische Therapie als "Übertragungsraum" in der Behandlung von Geflüchteten. Einige Bemerkungen zur Behandlungstechnik. In R. Haubl & H.-J. Wirth (Hrsg.), *Grenzerfahrungen* (pp. 219–234). Gießen: Psychosozialverlag.

Čunović, Ž., & Vukmanic, M. (2000). Lebens- und Behandlungsperspektiven traumatisierter bosnischer Flüchtlinge in Deutschland. *Psychoanalyse im Widerspruch, 23,* 65–77.

Kluge, U., & Kassim, N. (2006). Der Dritte im Raum. Chancen und Schwierigkeiten in der Zusammenarbeit mit Sprach- und Kulturmittlern in einem interkulturellen psychotherapeutischen Setting. In E. Wohlfart & M. Zaumseil (Eds.), *Transkulturelle Psychiatrie – Interkulturelle Psychotherapie*. Berlin, Heidelberg: Springer.

Laub, D., & Auerhahn, N. C. (1993). Knowing and not knowing massive psychic trauma: Forms of traumatic memory. *International Journal of Psychoanalysis, 74*(2), 287–302.

Leuzinger-Bohleber, M., & Hettich, N. (2018). What and how can psychoanalysis contribute in support of refugees? Concepts, clinical experiences and applications in the project STEP-BY-STEP, a pilot project supporting refugees in the initial reception center "Michaelisdorf" (Michaelis-village) in Darmstadt, Germany. *International Journal of Applied Psychoanalytic Studies, 15*(3), 151–173. doi:10.1002/aps.1584.

Leuzinger-Bohleber, M., Rickmeyer, C., Tahiri, M., Hettich, N., & Fischmann, T. (2016). What can psychoanalysis contribute to the current refugee crisis? *The International Journal of Psychoanalysis, 97*(4), 1077–1093. doi:10.1111/1745–8315.12542.

Miller, K. E., Martell, Z. L., Pazdirek, L., Caruth, M., & Lopez, D. (2005). The role of interpreters in psychotherapy with refugees: An exploratory study. *American Journal of Orthopsychiatry, 75*(1), 27–39. doi:10.1037/0002–9432.75.1.27.

Plänkers, T., Laier, M., Otto, H. H., Rothe, H. J., & Siefert, H. (1996). Psychoanalyse in Frankfurt am Main. In *Zerstörte Anfänge. Wiederannährung. Entwicklungen.* Tübingen: Brandes & Apsel.

Scheifele, S. (2021). Innen und Außen – Zum analytischen Raum in Psychotherapien mit Menschen, die aus ihrer Heimat geflohen sind. In L. Bayer & H. Weiß (Eds.), *Die Psychoanalytische Ambulanz Aufgaben und Arbeitsweisen am Beispiel des Sigmund-Freud-Instituts* (pp. 142–177). Stuttgart: Kohlhammer.

Sturm, E. (2018) Strukturen der Strukturverluste: Zur Entwicklung eines Behandlungsangebotes in der International Clinic des Frankfurter Psychoanalytischen Instituts. In *DPV-Tagungsband: "Übertragung, Szene, Mikroprozesse"* (pp. 319–329). Gießen: Psychosozial-Verlag.

Wohlfart, E., Özbek, T., & Heinz, A. (2005). *Von kultureller Antizipation zu transkulturellem Verstehen*. In H. J. Assion (Eds.), *Migration und seelische gesundheit*. Berlin, Heidelberg: Springer.

3 Forced to flee

The experience of Peruvian women in times of political violence[1]

Elizabeth Haworth

Psychoanalysis and migration

Most of the psychoanalytic literature on migration, since Grinberg and Grinberg,[2] has stressed the role of loss and mourning. They point out that migratory process goes through several phases:

i)   Intense sorrow for all that has been lost, fear of the unknown and deep experiences of loneliness, and helplessness (paranoid, confusion, and depressive anxieties).
ii) Manic state: the immigrant minimises the significance of the change in his or her life and overvalues everything new, disdaining what was in the past and lost.
iii) After a time, nostalgia appears as well as sorrow for the lost world. The person begins to recognise feelings previously dissociated or denied and is more accessible to incorporate elements of the new culture.
iv) Recovery of the pleasure of thinking and desiring to make plans for the future in which the past is regarded as such and not as a "lost paradise" where one constantly longs to return.

Varvin (2005)[3] states that trauma is a complex event occurring beyond normal horizons. Though it is defined retrospectively and has an effect on development, it is now considered a developmental disturbance in itself. He stresses the strong feelings of shame and somatic reactions to severe trauma. Extreme experiences will affect individuals and/or groups depending on the severity, complexity, and duration of traumatising events, as well as on context, developmental stage, and internal object relations. Furthermore, Varvin concludes, it will depend upon the extent to which earlier traumatic associations are activated.[4] Now, terror has many facets and a great potential for violence. Dictatorial regimes can take systematic steps to remove undesirable elements. The political ideological religious justifications represent a mental instrument that validate dehumanising the chosen enemy, giving meaning to the apparent necessity of exterminating undesirable, dangerous, or harmful elements in a battle between good and bad.

DOI: 10.4324/9781003203223-5

On the other hand, Rozmarin[5] postulates that psychoanalysis is a clinical practice and a theory of the human condition as well. Thus, immigration is a reality that involves our lives and our practices. It is a metaphor for something much more general, the unsettledness, otherness, and precarity that is part of the experience of being human. However, psychoanalysts continue to think and practice under the presumption that the most important happens in the nuclear family, and when contents beyond the domestic realm are reached, our concepts grow weak as well as our sense of legitimacy.

In the same line, Csillag[6] points out that sometimes migrants want to leave malignant and sinister environments. Following (Cerdin and Duboloy (2004),[7] she says that a life in a different, strange land can provide an opportunity for the revision of personal history and the possibility of repairing a damaged childhood. Thus, in some cases, immigration can facilitate healing and the development of a potential space in which to develop the capacity to think and build linkages.

Forced migration implies an uprooting that people experience as imposed by external conditions, but it is also an opportunity for new encounters and an attempt to solve previous conflicts. Clearly, forced migration implies a sort of coercion but also involves a decision for change and an illusion of improving women's lives. In this sense, there is an element of agency that is often overlooked in the discussions.

Internal migration in Peru

In order to understand the complexity of forced internal migration in the case of Peruvian women, we will present three points: i) the sudden transition from mothers to heads of household, ii) past and present violence, iii) the transgenerational impact in the daughters of migrants.

The sources used are a) the Report by the Commission of Truth and Reconciliation (CTR) submitted in 2002, which collected 12,000 testimonies; b) cases from the Centro de Atención Psicosocial (CAPS), which was one of the civil society organisations in charge of the legal and psychoanalytical care of cases of torture and political violence; c) a qualitative research study on the object relationships of women who migrated from Ayacucho to Lima when they were children due to the IAC.[8]

I will begin by describing some of the elements of the Peruvian context that may allow us to understand migration, violence, and women's social imaginaries.

Representational context: migration, violence, and women in Peru

Migration is a constitutive element of the history of Peru, marked by various internal displacements. The colonisation strategy of the Inca Empire forced displacements of entire ethnic groups. External migrations, such as the Spanish conquest and later ones, configured a *mestizo* identity.[9]

We must consider that Peru and Mexico were the most important Spanish viceroyalties in America, and Lima was the capital of the viceroyalty, establishing itself as a court society, with particular characteristics, attitudes that can be seen to this day. The process of independence with Spain did not imply that the differences between Indians and *criollos* (Creoles) were overcome, since that division prevails even today. Lima still holds the power, ignoring the rest of the country.

In order to understand women's participation in these processes, we must remember the various referents of being a woman in Peru. In the pre-Inca worldview, there are two important female deities: Mama Waco and Mama Ocllo. Mama Waco is a warrior, cruel and efficient. Mama Ocllo is the prototype of the nurturing mother. *"We were poor but she (my mother) always took care of us, of my siblings and me, she gave us affection. . . . [S]he hugged us and when she punished us, she also hit us hard."*[10] In this case, we observe how these models of care coexist through hugs and physical punishment. Women can be gentle and violent at the same time.

Obviously, these are not the only two referents Peruvian women have. The conquest fractured the community life organisation of the Tawantinsuyo, imposing Catholic religion, by the process of extirpation of idolatries and bringing a different vision of the relationship between men and women. Virgin Mary coexisted with the previous female deities.

Migrations in the last century

In the 20th century, two important internal displacements occurred from the provinces towards Lima: the so-called *population overflow* in the mid-1950s that continued until the 1960s, and the one forced by the internal armed conflict (IAC) in the 1980s. The first was generated by the change in economic patterns, the state of abandonment in which the provinces found themselves, and the need for basic rights. Lima was transformed from a semi viceroyal city to a provincial, colourful, and more *mestizo* capital.

This first migratory wave of the 20th century was part of collective projects framed in family and provincial networks of entrepreneurs and settlers in which women occupied urban lands, leading to the emergence of organisations that transformed the social and political life of the country. Men and women participated jointly in a common project of occupying the capital in search of a better future. Women decided to come; in many cases, they were the engines of the migratory project; they had agency. This led to an increase of awareness of their rights, especially among the next generation.

The IAC that affected Peru since 1980 and up until 2000 caused 69,280 deaths and over 500,000 displacements, provoking a social fracture still pending to understand and solve. During these years, a paranoid feeling was experienced in cities where there were organisations, and actions that expressed distrust were generated: installing fences or railings in dwellings; in streets, limiting exchanges in public spaces. The others, including policemen, could be a threat. The IAC entailed a traumatised mass of people, mainly women and children, who ran to the capitals of provinces and to Lima to escape from the violence, with an uncertain destination.

In both cases, with the internal migration, the Creole fear of an *Indian invasion* re-emerged. For many people in Lima, as a result of centralism and discrimination, migrants from the mountains were foreigners, with different customs; they were not understood and were rejected. Internal parts of oneself as Indians were rejected and projected on the others. We can be reminded of Julia Kristeva: *The lesson of the foreigner is that we all are foreigners, not only before strangers but above all before ourselves.*[11]

The sudden transition from mothers to heads of household

We share a scene that unfortunately became commonplace:

> *This morning the soldiers rounded up the people of Nuevo Occoro, they gathered all the people in the square, there were around 100 people including men, children, women and older people. In the square, the soldiers separated men and women; the latter were placed in the town hall, and they did not let them move. When they came to the square, they made the men squat. . . . [T]hey hit them and took them away. . . . [F]rom that date nothing was known about them.*[12]

One aspect of this scene we wish to highlight is the place of women. While men received direct physical aggression, women were confined, locked, and forced to accuse men of their community. In other cases, they received direct aggressions, such as sexual violence and humiliation and insults when they were searching for their disappeared relatives. During and after the conflict, women had to become actively involved in the processes of search and claim for justice, being subject to abuse, ill-treatment, sexual harassment, rape, torture, displacement, and forced migration. Women had to face alone a new context under violent and sudden conditions. In addition, they had to oversee the survival of their family, leading emergency departures from the communities towards peripheral locations, such as urban centres nearby and capitals of provinces. All these circumstances demanded a great capacity of adaptation and over-adaptation that affected their physical and mental health.

> *It was hell for us, we were no longer happy, losing a father was sad. [T]here was fear. Sometimes hens would be frightened around there, we would run*

> *away. Sometimes dogs barked around here, we were running away because of fear, we could no longer sleep or eat or sit down calmly. Nothing any longer.*

We see how fear, terror is installed, and it does not go away. The allusion to *Ilakis* in several interviews – a Quechua word that alludes to painful thoughts and memories that reach the heart, the place where painful emotions rest – is found in many testimonies of women who were witnesses of violence. The traumatic scenes return over and over with much clarity and horror, also for those who listen to them. The anxiety of death, the sensation of loneliness, and the experience of permanent madness accompanied many of these women. They could not, we could not, understand the reason for this violence. The magnitude of the events made the efforts of civil society as well as the state insufficient to attend the population.

Although in both migrations, women played an important role, in that provoked by the IAC, the community fabric was torn; women were alone and had to rebuild, not always successfully, new groups that would somehow substitute those lost.

An interesting aspect of this change is that it represented moving away from stereotypical male and female roles. These psychic dynamics and changes in gender roles established new foundations in this continuous process of restoration and a new social construction after the uprooting.

Transgenerational impact of violence on the daughters of women who lived through the internal armed conflict

The following vignettes are taken from qualitative research on object relationships of women who migrated during IAC, using the Thematic Apperception Test (TAT). In this case, we present some of the interviews made to the daughters of the migrant women.

> *I have the image of her being aware if I leave well sheltered, that I have my clothes in order and that I eat well. . . . [T]hey are many beautiful memories because at that time I was a girl and I always had her by my side, a person who does your stuff, who takes care of you, cares about you.*
>
> (FM1 – Fernanda, November 2012)

> *[M]mm . . . they are beautiful memories when I was little and your mom protects you and takes care of you and everything. . . . I remember as a little girl living in my grandparents' house, they were always super workers, both . . . and my mom also doing everything.*

In these two interviews, it is appreciated how the mother is perceived as the main care figure. These mothers have been able to preserve in their daughters the idea of a beautiful world despite the tragedy experienced.

They would play a mediating role in preventing impingement. In the daughters, in turn, a splitting mechanism could be produced to preserve a good object and project the negative in the absent father. This idealised image of the mother is socially influenced by society (religion, Virgin Mary).

> [Y]es, I remember that they separated, but I think . . . I really do not know how it was. My father worked his land and at that time because of terrorism, they captured people and took him or killed him. . . . [W]hen I was a little older, my mother told me that he, my father, had to run. . . . [H]e abandoned us, but I do not know what happened to him, if he is still alive. . . . I do not know anything.
>
> *(GG2 – Gina, November 2012)*

The father is an enigmatic figure; she does not know if he's alive or dead, if he left by his own will or by obligation. The figure of the father is a void that generates anguish in the mother. This will be important for the future development of women and their subjective perception of the feminine. In the social imaginary, the mothers are the strong women, those who face the problems, they are affectionate and, at the same time, hard. Fathers are more absent, perceived as weaker, require protection, and emotionally opaque. This could suggest a problem in identifying with the masculine/active aspect.

> Well, what I see is that suddenly an earthquake has occurred, a disaster and you may be sad, no? Because of a relative, thinking that now you have lost a relative and you have been left alone. You must go on forward while you are alive.
>
> *(GG2 – Gina, November 2012)*

This reference to the fact that they lived an earthquake[13] is quite frequent among those who lived through the IAC. As girls, they lived the earthquake lived by their relatives. The simile has to do with the sudden, the destructiveness, the loss of continuity with no possible escape, only taking defensive measures – therefore, a traumatic experience. This accounts for how alien the causes of the conflict were for the population who suffered it, the absence of information made it more unintelligible. *Going forward* could be a forward defence, but also a creative search for a solution, recognising that they still have a life.

Migration from Venezuela

Since 2000, concerned about the uncertain economic situation in their country, Venezuelans started to migrate. The second wave started around

2012 with the end of the oil and mineral commodities boom in Latin America, deepening the economic crisis, political repression, and food and medicines shortages. They migrated to regional countries as Colombia and Peru. Peru granted temporary work permits (PPT) that allowed them to work. The last wave followed the death of Hugo Chávez and the election of Nicolás Maduro in 2013, in a context where social, political, and economic conditions worsened considerably, creating a humanitarian crisis. Migrants in this wave came from diverse demographic backgrounds.

We rely on information recollected in a study with migrant women workers from CARE PERU and IDEHPUCP[14] and in some interviews with migrant women. We think that the comparison with internal migration in Peru can shed some light on the particularities of migration according to gender within the region.

In the survey carried out by CARE and IDEHPUCP, it was identified that 78.8% of the women had entered the country in the last two years (2018–2019). They said they migrated due to economic difficulties in Venezuela, the shortage of food and medicine, social and political conditions, or the need to reconnect with their relatives. This is a first difference with men's migration. Women usually have family behind or in the receptor country that depend on them.

The women interviewed indicated that they had a good reception during the first months of arrival, but, soon, the attitude of Peruvian people changed.

> *There is a negative perception about Venezuelan citizens. I have seen this in restaurants, sometimes; they do not accept that you are a foreigner. In the same rentals, they don't allow you to stay. It is a sad thing then, because you want to work but when you see that kind of behavior, everything becomes difficult.*
>
> (Migrant woman, Trujillo, 29 years old)

One of the main differences with inner migration is that most Venezuelan women have better educational and labour skills. Unfortunately, not all of them could work on their previous jobs, having to adapt to care jobs as domestic services with all the disadvantages and particularities it has in Peruvian society. Domestic service is one of the most informal jobs in Peru, with no written contract and in private residences, thus with no possibility of regulation from the state. Most of the women work in hard conditions, although in the last years, many of them have increased their salaries. Anyway, discrimination and racism continue unaltered, and this is a scenario unfamiliar to new migrants:

> *We agreed to work 8 hours, but in the end, I worked 10 or more. I had to take care of a baby and at the end, I was in charge of the entire house. My salary*

was supposed to be paid on the 25th but it was the end of the month, and I didn't receive my payment. I think they (Peruvians) *treat their own people very bad.*

There is a cultural difference we are taught to obey but not to be masochistic. We do not speak in a bad way, but we do know how to say it. Look, what they tell us to do, we do, in the best way, with a good face. We work on what they tell us, but if they are going to humiliate us, we respond. We tell the same person up front.

(Migrant woman, 37 years old)

Another big difference is how Venezuelan women are more concerned with their body and appearance. Years before, they were admired by local women and men, but now they are perceived with distrust and even envy, provoking hostile responses in women and men as well.

They see us as prostitutes; the men in the streets come up to us and say "Hey Veneca, let's have sex." Another woman said: *They chase me when I get off the bus, they chase me to my house, men come outside my work and say ugly things to me.*

This situation is worsened by the way the media depicts Venezuelans as criminals and women as prostitutes. This has changed in the last political campaign as they were used against one of the candidates accused of being a communist. Venezuelans then changed to *brothers and sisters in the struggle for democracy.*

To continue thinking

Internal migrations in Peru in the 20th century have meant not only changes in families and in male and female relationships, but also internal displacements that re-signify inner self images and relations that need further research. The same is occurring with Venezuelan migration.

In the case of internal migration of Peruvian women, the influence of internal displacement by the IAC in the female subjectivity requires further investigation. From research and social movements, we see a split between an image of *brave, empowered women, mothers-fathers, and suffering victims, mothers* (always). The community bond was broken by violence and years later by the neoliberal economic model, weakening the possibility of creating collectives and disempowering women.

The period of violence mobilised civil society and the state. It was a moment of great effervescence and impact that, in some way, allowed a social reunification, although with limitations. However, we can see that the historical social fracture was sharpened.

There are two aspects we would like to highlight: i) the appearance of gangs of adolescent women, particularly in Ayacucho after the IAC whose violence is discharged without a clear object, showing the dramatic effects of this period; and ii) currently, femicides in Peru, one of the highest numbers in LA. Due to the characteristics of some of them, we can ask how much territorial **and** internal displacement is implicated in the relations between men and women. It is an issue to be investigated that would give more light to understand the relations between men and women associated with the feminist movements that have also been very influential in the country and in the region.

In the case of Venezuelan migrants, there is a good deal of research to be done. We still need to focus on how migration is affecting the subjectivity of men, women, and especially children. The pandemic has had an impact on all of us that still needs to be examined in depth. The work that is being done by psychologists and psychoanalysts as CAPS will highlight these issues. One thing is for sure; Venezuelan migration, as internal migration did at its time, will change Peru's social dynamics.

Notes

1 I would like to thank Cecilia Martínez and Rocío Franco, psychoanalysts of the Peruvian Psychoanalytic Society and co-members of the Zuno group. We have been working for more than 20 years in bringing psychoanalysis to other social fields.
2 Grinberg, L., & Grinberg, R. (1984). A psychoanalytic study of migration: It's normal and pathological aspects. *Journal of the American Psychoanalytic Association, 32,* 13–38.
3 Varvin, S. (2005). Humiliation and the victim identity in conditions of political and violent conflict. *Scandinavian Psychoanalytic Review, 28*(1), 40–49.
4 Varvin, S. (2017). Our relations to refugees: Between compassion and dehumanization. *American Journal of Psychoanalysis, 77*(4), 359.
5 Rozmarin, E. (2017). Immigration, belonging, and the tension between center and margin in *psychoanalysis. Psychoanalytic Dialogues, 27*(4), 470–479.
6 Csillag, V. (2017). Emmy grant: Immigration as repetition of trauma and a potential space. *Psychoanalytic Dialogues, 27*(4), 454–469.
7 Cerdin, J., & Duboloy, M. (2004). Expatriation as a maturational opportunity: A psychoanalytic approach based on "copy and paste." *Human Relations, 57*(8), 957–982.
8 Llerena, L. (2014). *Relaciones objétales: estudio cualitativo con mujeres desplazadas por el conflicto armado en el Peru.* Bachelor Thesis in Psychology, Universidad Peruana de Ciencias Aplicadas, Lima, Peru.
9 Throughout its history, Peru has received migrants from Spain (the colonizers), Africa (the slaves), China, Japan, and Italy, and in recent years, from Venezuela.
10 Gina, interview, op. cit. p. 49.
11 Kristeva, J. (1991). *Strangers to ourselves.* New York, NY: Columbia University Press.
12 Report of the Truth and Reconciliation Commission, p. 163.
13 Peru is located in the Pacific Ring of Fire, which is a seismic zone where tremors and earthquakes are frequent.
14 CARE PERU and Instituto de Democracia y Derechos Humanos de la Pontificia Universidad Católica del Peru (IDEHPUCP). (2020, Agosto). *Las mujeres migrantes y refugiadas venezolanas y su inserción en el mercado laboral peruano: dificultades, expectativas y potencialidades.* Lima: CARE PERU and IDEHPUCP.

4 Perinatal migration

Lived experience and intergenerational transmission

Joan Raphael-Leff

The need for personal recognition is at the heart of our human condition. But a migrant can no longer take for granted being known or knowing. This has implications for pregnancy and confidence in mothering.

This chapter draws on my half century of specialisation in reproductive issues. In addition to clinical work and workshops/focus groups with expectant/parents, I have served as consultant to perinatal services in over 40 countries, providing teaching, training, and clinical supervision to professional therapists, lay practitioners, counsellors, primary health carers, midwives, health visitors, and so on in groups and/or individually (usually through interpreters). Programmes differ in setting, venue, and content of their provisions from bare minimum to ongoing home visits; from a one-off meeting to ongoing help; before, during and/or after the birth; from open-ended to theme-based sessions in group, individual, or family sessions; conducted in baby clinics or detention centres; or in home visits to township shacks, city dwellings, or more affluent suburbia. Some projects focus specifically on migrants; others are inclusive, screening all local childbearing women, including those from elsewhere. But in common, these innovative ventures (usually run by non-profit NGOs) aim to reduce emotional distress, while promoting physical safety.

It is noteworthy that cross-cultural work or that in multiethnic societies raises epistemological issues about imposing our own theoretical framework, values, and tacit assumptions on others in the context of language barriers, cultural differences, and hierarchical power structures.

Crucially, crossing geographical boundaries affects a childbearing woman's fundamental sense of security. Studies estimate that one in three migrants develop a diagnosable perinatal mental illness during pregnancy or early motherhood (compared to 13%–20% of settled women in the same locality). Emotional states are compounded by posttraumatic stress with involuntary flashbacks to recent unspeakable events. Given the heterogenous conditions of migration – the nature of flight, privations of the journey, and hardships in the new destination – a variety of intersecting variables of social disadvantage combine in different ways. These influence each woman's approach to the tribulations of pregnancy and

DOI: 10.4324/9781003203223-6

motherhood and are likely to impact on her ability to negotiate the complexities of accessing health services in a foreign country.

Perinatal susceptibility

Pregnancy and early motherhood are known to be periods of great vulnerability. Even in stable populations, parental disorders are very common during the thousand days from conception until age two. My research indicates that disruption is often precipitated by a salient trigger during pregnancy or particular developmental stage of the baby that reactivates preconscious residues of painful ordeals which can impact on a mother's receptivity to her infant and/or may become re-enacted interactively within the dyad. The nature and timing of emotional disturbance usually reflect *the weakest links* of the adult's own infancy or childhood (Raphael-Leff, 2017). Disturbance ranges from antenatal to postnatal, mild to acute, and passing or chronic and may be accompanied by breakthrough representations of unprocessed violations or neglect, Numerous studies find that childhood adversity results in up to a twelvefold increase in alcoholism, drug dependency, and self-harm later in life. Severe conditions during pregnancy may have a direct hormonal effect on the unborn child implicated in impaired neurodevelopment and potential behavioural problems (see Monk et al., 2020).[1]

While attention is often paid to postnatal depression, perinatal disorders can be multifactorial, including persecutory disorders such as paranoia, phobias, obsessive-compulsive syndromes, and rarely, postpartum psychosis. For instance, findings show that some 20%–40% of depressed mothers also report obsessional thoughts of harming the child. Alarmingly, in societies where childbirth mortality is decreased, suicide is now a leading cause of maternal death, sometimes accompanied by infanticide.

Numerous studies cite ongoing challenges that aggravate the emotional condition. These include poverty, gender inequalities, domestic violence, physical illnesses, complications of childbirth, the stresses of childcare, and increasingly, internal displacement and migration. Recurrently mentioned are two protective factors in a childbearing individual's capacity to withstand major life events – *personal resilience* and *social support*.

In many societies, *young* mothers are particularly vulnerable. Teens encounter more complications in childbirth due to pelvic-cephalic disproportion and high rates of STDs. Levels of distress are raised when the physiological turmoil of pregnancy coincides with pubertal bodily changes, clashing emotional demands of a pressing desire for self-actualisation and commitment to a dependent baby.

Unsurprisingly, young mothers have a *threefold rate of postnatal disturbance* during the storm and stress of adolescence, exacerbated by physical and emotional immaturity, as well as potentially destructive intergenerational sexual relationships, while coping simultaneously with these two major transitional upheavals. Practitioners are often critical of surging passions in young parents; however, teenage separation-individuation conflicts are intensified when confronted by similar bids for independence in their toddlers (Raphael-Leff, 2012).

Whatever parental age, throughout the world, perinatal emotional distress is heightened by precipitants such as rape, transactional sex, or a history of child sexual abuse. Environmental provisions are crucial too. Unwanted conception prevails in locations with lower access to female contraception and safe abortion (not only in far-off "non-developed" countries but within moralistic states of the USA!). Mental ill-health during pregnancy and following childbirth is clearly linked to geo-economic factors. Prevalence is twice to thrice higher in low-income countries (where over 90% of the worlds' babies are born).[2] One reason for this discrepancy is a drastic fall in earnings. Most high-income societies offer paid maternity leave. Scandinavia and the Nordic countries are especially generous, with paternal leave too, and ongoing psychological support until the youngest child goes to school. That said, even in prosperous societies, migrants and local black and minority (BME) communities tend to fare worse, as discriminatory aspects of ethnicity, culture, language, and gender intersect with mental health. This discrepancy has long-lasting effects. One large British study (AESOP) found that migration, coupled with social isolation, unemployment, and achievement-expectation mismatch considerably raised the rates of first episode psychosis, *even in second- and third-generation ethnic minorities* (Morgan & Hutchinson, 2010).

Recently, greater awareness of BME perinatal issues is specifically addressed in a UK government report, calling for better pre- and post-registration training to strengthen practitioners' culturally sensitive understanding and to develop/improve commissioning and service-provision and care pathways to meet the needs of *all* women, including migrants (www.gov.uk/government/publications/national-perinatal-mental-health-project-report).

Perinatal migration

Most migrants experience a triple trauma – *displacement* and loss of forbearers (traditions, material possessions, ancestral graves, primal voices); *transition* – suffering a disequilibrium of impermanence, risks, and possible loss of family members in the crossing; *arrival* – with new demands of acclimatisation and acculturation.

Loss of motherland is especially salient for a woman undertaking motherhood in a new location. Involuntary dislocation massively increases the risk of perinatal disturbance. The most fundamental sense of security and constancy are eroded when home is abandoned in fear. Severance from her archaic sensory backdrop means losing touch with her subsymbolic experience such as tacit rhythms of wake, sleep, and feeding; implicit voices of encouragement or scolding.

Clearly, a great difference exists between emergency migration – taking few tangible mementoes and leaving behind a wrecked or erased history – and one of embarking on a journey, however tortuous, emboldened by ideology or hope of bettering one's family fortune. However, irrespective of whether departure was chosen or enforced, on an unconscious level, *leaving behind the land of one's birth entails physical disconnection from primary* sensual *anchors, familiar landmarks, and temporality.*

Living elsewhere, predictability is affected by severance from implicit knowability of seasonal changes. Migration fractures links with sites and festive celebrations, with familiar foods and vegetation; the subliminal minutiae of home comfort and social custom – recurrent rituals, local music scales, intoxicating odours and everyday noises, colourful fabrics, and unforgettable tastes of smoky or honey-soaked street foods . . . and the melodious lilt of lullabies and childhood chanting games – all deeply inscribed yet painfully beyond reach.

In contemporary globalisation, migration to Europe has accelerated in speed and scale. London is an example of a multiethnic city where over 300 languages are now spoken. Around the world, in addition to exile or flight from situations of war, poverty, prejudice, rape, and/or torture, climate change now forces people to flee their homeland due to drought, famine, and floods. Whether overland by foot, cart, or vehicle, or in over-crowded boats, travellers often endure long periods of danger, risking re-traumatisation. Stressors differ with rural-to-urban or cross-border migration and whether the incentive is economic, religious, or political.

But in common, within a fragmented, disintegrating world, *trust in stability is eroded.*

People living in an unfamiliar location often encounter ordeals of xenophobia. Homelessness renders them susceptible to being "othered." Economic migrants, refugees, and exiled asylum seekers are disproportionately exposed to discrimination and prejudice, intimidation, and in some situations, actual physical attacks.

Over half of the world's refugees are children, many separated from their families.[3]

Additionally, lowered resistance and lack of immunity to local infections renders migrants extra vulnerable to illness and disease. Findings show a higher prevalence of asthma and food allergies in both transient and adopted countries compared to their countries of origin.

Displaced pregnant women and new mothers are especially susceptible. Ill-health, poor diet, and lack of adequate nourishment impinge on the unborn baby's development, also affect breastfeeding. Maternal emotional disturbance in pregnancy also has further implications for the unborn child: low birth weight and preterm delivery associated with poor antenatal clinic attendance. Unfamiliar birth-giving practices are a further obstacle. Disposal of the umbilical cord and afterbirth may cause additional distress when ceremonial burial or diet-enriching ingestion is prevented. For women from countries where FGM is prevalent, birth may involve humiliation from shocked and bewildered Western midwives unfamiliar with the ramifications of genital infibulations.

Furthermore, worldwide, depression, persecution, anxiety, and childhood abuse are associated with maternal self-harm, such as alcohol and substance abuse and risk-taking behaviours, including enactments and unhealthy lifestyles, smoking, poor diet, self-medication, and cutting. For migrants, additional factors such as social isolation and language difficulties compound side-effects of perinatal depression and anxiety, further decreasing maternal initiative to seek out well-baby clinics and advice about vaccination, family planning, and so on.

Perinatal identity, defences, and bonding

A pregnant woman's familiar sense of self is often undermined by rapid biochemical and physiological changes. Being assailed by the somatic and psychological impact of powerful birth experiences in an alienating hospital environment undermines identity, as a parturient's previous lifestyle feels overwhelmed by the life-and-death demands of her new role.

In recent times, security has further decreased with geographical mobility, whether disaster driven, for economic betterment, or political refuge. The UN put the 2019 figure for people displaced from their homes by war, conflict, and persecution at *71 million*! More than 25 million of these are refugees, having fled across international borders and unable to return to their homes.

Hannah Arendt said after World War II that refugees suffer a double loss – of self and of a common world. As she understood, when migrants lack the "Right to Have Rights," *powerlessness* becomes "the major experience of their lives" (Arendt, 1998, p. 237).

Yet even when a hospitable country offers relative safety, a childbearing migrant is taking a leap into the unknown. However welcoming or idealised the host country, local parenting patterns can still seem incongruous and strange. She is inserting roots into foreign soil. Her child's world will differ from her own. She will take for granted regulative concessions and constraints of which the mother is ignorant. While struggling to reconstitute her shattered life in this place, a mother strives to learn new ways even while hoping to pass on old family traditions to her child.

Antenatal bonding is adversely affected when the pregnancy is laden not only with the usual investment of aspirations, dreams, and desires, but carries extra emotional significance – a replacement baby to compensate for other losses, the fatherless child of a deceased partner. Specific difficulties arise in forming a positive connection with a baby conceived in hatred, who will be a constant reminder of a horrible ordeal of non-consensual sex, gang rape, even torture.

A migrant mother often lacks a caregiving buffer. When her own sense of deprivation and childhood grievance surface, competitiveness may be rife. As defence structures crumble, impulses of punitive vengeance may erupt, with possible projection of malevolence onto the infant who becomes a repository of ancient or more recent experiences of aggression or abuse. Lacking emotional support, mothers often buckle under the strain.

As psychoanalysts, we are well aware of the deleterious long-term emotional consequences of stress and high maternal anxiety for an impressionable infant.

In common, those arriving from elsewhere live with the complexities of acculturation and a sense of dual temporality – frozen time past and urgent present time. To many, a sense of alienation is retained from the migratory experience itself. In addition to maternal exhaustion and deprivation of dream sleep, an isolated migrant may have no one to converse with intimately.

Some are weighed down by after-effects of a harrowing journey and remain burdened by unprocessed experiences of the original dispossession.

If ejection from her native soil involved horrendous scenes of aggression and brutality, a heavy-duty mental defence may have been employed – strong enough to block the intolerable imagery of unspeakable horrors etched on the retina and unheralded flashbacks of mindless terror that tear into sleepless nights in a strange bed in a foreign land.

Dissociation is one such survival mechanism that allows people to endure traumatic experiences of violence and unbearable pain of loss.

Many migrant mothers have, of necessity, resorted to a pattern of defensive blocking in reaction to trauma. But detachment, defeatism, or apathy also increase the strain in summoning enough emotional energy to rejoice in a pregnancy so overshadowed by suffering, loss of faraway loved ones, and cherished places seen for the last time.

In addition, daily life often remains precarious, with financial shortage and social embarrassment. Maternal emotional disconnection may also be accompanied by suspiciousness and hypervigilance to change in a world where acceptance is conditional with few and indefinite opportunities for perfectibility. But her constant alertness to potential danger with states of mind at variance with emotional availability for reflective functioning engenders a traumatic attachment (Moore, 2022).[4]

Communication is crucial, but a migrant mother is often bereft of extended community of easy amicability with known people with whom she shares a common language and lifestyle. Multiple absences of family members and friends compounded by the lack of someone from back home with whom she shares childhood memories and maternal lore or even another migrant to compare her exilic standpoint. Even when she carries a treasure trove of cultural references, lacking a confidante, the isolated woman reels, dizzy with both disorientation and nostalgia.

On a practical level, learning the lingo and opening a bank account may prove insurmountable obstacles for a mother who has other children to feed and clothe and/or lacks a guide. Little gestures of kindness can offer a glimpse of connection, a little flare of joy in a harsh existence. Conversely, the daily struggle just to keep going in the face of her losses may aggravate her reluctance to form new human contacts.

Often denied the right to work, her own skills go unappreciated. Like a toddler, she experiences a steep learning curve – having to relearn the shape and meaning of basic concepts. Uttering words that hurt her mouth to pronounce. Listening to different drumbeats, to language rhythms that puzzle as she struggles to identify one familiar word in a rush of gobble-dygook utterances.

As her identity contracts, she feels like a shadow of her former full-bodied passionate, even voluptuous, self – a non-citizen with no contribution to make. She may be highly qualified but lacks proof. Sometimes, if certificates and diplomas were lost in the move, she is refused recognition and has to retrain. Not knowing the rules also further undermines her personal strengths and recognised limitations. When she cannot express her thoughts for lack of a common language, she turns into an observer rather than a fully-fledged self-assured participant.

Perinatal "contagious arousal"

Nuzzling her floppy newborn, a new mother finds herself catapulted back into archaic perceptual channels and pre-reflective passions which engender intense anxiety in a vulnerable carer, especially in the absence of transgenerational mediation.

On the bus or in the street, walking among inscrutable people, jostled yet separate and apart, she feels an unknown stranger, both invisible and yet a target of evasion or even hostility. She disciplines herself to a cautious existence – not too loud, not too prominent, not too obvious – a tension between submission and defeat. As well as awareness of fierce competition over the basic essentials of survival.

Forfeiture of her familial protective "bubble" inclines a migrant mother to shield her swollen belly or defenceless child from unresponsive glances or inquisitive stares of strangers. But caution may also lead to rejection of unfamiliar baby-care advice or well-intentioned offers of assistance. Unsurprisingly, when the carapace cracks, florid symptoms may erupt.

Loss of the matrix

Early parenthood is always a time of intense provocation. Our primary form of sensory representation is acquired by being parented in infancy.

In adulthood, the textures, sounds, smells, and feel of a neonate reactivate implicit substrates of our own preverbal babyhoods. Today, many Westernised parents are unfamiliar with babies and unprepared for the emotional impact on their lives of a tiny tot. People who parent together bring the unremembered experience of their own respective infancies – which may or may not harmonise. This organisational framework of childbearing partners includes not only their own preconscious relational representations but multilayered transgenerational introjections and unconscious sediments from their own parents' parenting histories. When they come from elsewhere, an isolated couple's intimate relationship often fails under unrealistic expectations – a pressure to meet urgent demands that in their home country would have been distributed among several loving caregivers. In addition, stressors related to the migration process and to local social discrimination and exclusion impact on parental functioning.

Apart from migration, rapid urbanisation around the world has also resulted in dispersal of extended family networks and scarce conventions. Based on my clinical experience and cross-cultural consultancy, I argue that in more settled traditional societies (such as Norway), where generations follow established patterns of parenting, time and time again opportunities arise to work through infantile feelings with the birth of a sibling, cousin, or neighbour's baby, in the presence of containing adults, who later also offer guidance to mother and baby. Elsewhere, stratified societies-in-transition with small nuclear families offer little chance to safely process unresolved issues and feelings of confusion, frustration, and jealousy are commonly reactivated during pregnancy and early parenting in adults who have had little experience of young infants before becoming parents themselves.

Recent neuropsychological research notes that our representations during the first year of life before maturation of the hippocampus are encoded in a non-verbal, imagistic, acoustic, visceral, or temporal modes of information. This non-semantically encrypted experience remains stored in perceptual, sensorial, and imagistic channels.

To recap. I suggest that early parenting is troubling precisely because the sensual stimuli of baby-care intimately resemble conditions when the carer's own early experience was absorbed and thus encoded. I argue that because the very foundation of our parenting exists at a preverbal level, emotional arousal occurs when a parent is continuously having to interpret the infant's modes of expressiveness. It is subliminally reactivated through a process of *"contagious resonance"* as I've termed it, when the primary carer's own procedural experience is retriggered.

But, in addition, the new mother is in close contact with *primal substances* (eg, amniotic fluid, vernix, lochia, mucus, colostrum, breast milk, baby poop, pee, and posset). I argue that these potent effluences evoke *subsymbolic schema* (as Bucci called visceral, sensory, and somatic forms of representations (Bucci, 1997)). *Exposure to the smell and textures of primary substances elicit recall of the non-remembered past,* including subconsciously perceived emotions invested in her by her own archaic caregivers.

All this is disturbed in a strange environment.

On a social level, too, the baby can pose a threat. Not only are there unknown expectations of maternal behaviour, but her shortcomings risk becoming public simply by her baby yelling in the supermarket. Unconsciously, she also feels that the exacting infant who has been inside her and knows all her defects could disclose her hidden faults. Although this is a potential source of shame, the unruly child allows for vicarious expression for her own suppressed grief or prohibited "alien" facets affecting the child's own development of a sense of agency.

On the other hand, caution is called for in interpreting primary interaction, especially cross-culturally. Working with migrants involves respect for their own way of being, but also awareness that have experiences beyond our ken. We must open a dialogue. What may seem like provocation, cruel teasing, or overly strict discipline could be a maternal effort to "toughen" the child in preparation for inescapable racism or adverse circumstances of exclusion and destitution.

Therapeutic help to talk about and better understand her own feelings is invaluable when a mother feels distressed by unprocessed experience that is now becoming available to be articulated. Timely intervention can restore rapport with her baby, before the parent's incongruous response generates a distorted relational pattern.

Transcultural perinatal interventions

Although babies are a society's future, too few governments recognise the importance (and cost-effectiveness) of investing in the first 1,000 days between conception and two years. The process of persuasion has been slow.[5]

Growing evidence of the effect of perinatal emotional disturbances on both the suffering mother and her infant have galvanised mental health programmes to identify vulnerable pregnant women and/or mothers and offer some form of therapeutic intervention of counselling and/or psychiatric services (Field et al., 2014).[6] Meanwhile, determined to safeguard maternal well-being and/or infant mental health, various initiatives around the world, often set up by non-profit NGOs, feel compelled to step in to augment sparse or dysfunctional early years' provisions.

Even in this seemingly universal field, childbearing women have vastly different expectations and diverse experiences and a multitude of strongly held cultural beliefs about baby needs. As in all clinical work, it is essential to avoid imposing one's ideas and values. Awareness that one's own mindset is rooted in a particular epistemology helps to question the generalisability and transferability of our knowledge systems.

In multiethnic societies we therapists must develop a capacity to encompass manifold perspectives. This is essential in attempting to deliver culturally appropriate clinical interventions to newcomers and ethnic minorities in our own societies or in cross-cultural community mental health settings elsewhere.

Our taken-for-granted conventions are always already infused with social standards, power structures, identifications, and precepts of sexual difference and gender identity. In this intersecting narrative, our clients too, bring personal identifications and social norms, constraints and traditions intergenerationally transmitted in early relational contexts. Historically, this did not stop us Westerners from foisting our views on whole populations to the point of marginalising traditional beliefs and eliminating local methods of healing and welfare.

Today, we strive for *a dialogue* to become aware of each of our clients' own normative beliefs and ways to incorporate them (eg, interface theory assumes a possible complementarity). But while exploring strategies for incorporation of indigenous childcare beliefs alongside mainstream health care, we also must be alert to potential misunderstandings.[7]

In my own work as advisor or supervisor, my thinking is primarily psychoanalytic, but I am conscious that its application must be shaped by current needs and cultural, regional, environmental, even seasonal variations and local parameters. Focus-group discussion can clarify such priorities.

For instance, where clients cannot cover the cost of travel expenses and a single session is all that is feasible, the prime question is how to maximise the effect of that brief precious time together such that it can be utilised when the mother is on her own with her baby. Realistic planning must admit the emotional complexity and practical difficulties of mothering ahead.

Simply formulated: *what can this woman take away to help her make best use of her own potential resources?* We trust that good rapport in the single available session may encourage her to take advantage of telephone contact in the future.

Likewise, we know that focusing together in the session on what is "hot" can lessen the risk of malign enactments at home. But in low-income settings, the hottest priority is food, shelter, and safety. A common question is how one provides therapy to a homeless mother or a migrant whose shack has been burnt down by xenophobic neighbours? Working in subsistence economies, many counsellors admit that despite knowing this crosses therapeutic boundaries, they have given impoverished clients money, food, or baby clothes – asking how a hungry woman could be satisfied with mere words. They have a valid point. But sadly, funding constraints usually mean that few projects can afford to subsidise meagre national provisions.

In my experience, one starting point to foster the best use of even the most penurious client's inner strengths is by acknowledging *the importance of feelings* – her own feelings, and those of her (future) infant.

In common, pregnant women or new mothers may seek counsel in the hope of giving the baby more or better than they received, especially in the absence of maternal support. But many are also embroiled in their own childhood deprivations, envying their child's comparative privileges and resenting his or her demands on meagre resources. So, preparing the client to recognise the *inevitability of ambivalence* in all intimate relations is a valuable asset, especially when cultivating empathic understanding in meeting the baby's emotional needs.

These lessons can be important for the counsellors too, especially those who come from the same disadvantaged communities as their clients. Their work tends to stir their own feelings of guilt, grief, regret. Ironically, they may envy the understanding they themselves provide, conscious they did not have this luxury with their own babies. Therapists and counsellors offer a vital role model of reflective listening. But, as in all therapies, indeed, as in mothering – exposure to raw emotion which resonates with one's own personal history, interferes with remaining open to the other's pain. In addition to close identification and over-involvement, concrete thinking, emotional exhaustion, and depression are rife among lay counsellors with a high rate of burnout, especially among those who have experienced similar adverse life events as their clients (see Bain et al., 2019).

We assume that to avoid the high risk of practitioner fallout, their training is enhanced by awareness of their own subjective vulnerabilities. Emotional competence and a capacity to process their feelings increase through experiential groups, personal counselling, and peer support. Supervisory groups also enable counsellors to process their own unconscious projections, understand "countertransference," and to challenge their supervisors' cultural impositions, prompting them to modify their own theory.

Likewise, in working with migrants, a mainstream therapist may find it difficult to imagine, or indeed believe, the client's experience. Working through an interpreter adds an element of confusion, resulting in further distancing and simple questions like *"How many children do you have?"* or *"Who is the baby's father?"* may be loaded. Establishing therapeutic group work can validate extreme experience, sharing experiences while recognising that specificities differ.

In conclusion, I draw here on my own subjectivity. A long history of ancestral migration – generations criss-crossing Europe and beyond, fleeing prejudice, pogroms or holocaust, avoiding the Tsars' conscription, or seeking betterment, and daunting voyages leading to greater safety - or death.

Migrating from England to South Africa in 1918, the teenager who was to become my father was rescued from the North Sea when their ship, the *Galway Castle*, was torpedoed, and his mother and four sisters drowned. In 1949 my parents left Apartheid South Africa for Israel, and I myself left there in 1969 as a migrant of conscience.

Transgenerational influences prevail. Multilayered psychic richness often remains unspoken when crossing linguistic barriers and geographical boundaries. Rejecting yet absorbing projections of otherness, migrants live with both the precariousness and imaginative insights of marginality. Heightened generational gaps are marked by inspirational cross-pollination and yet estrangement. Children carry a burdensome yet triumphal role-reversal as savvy interpreters/negotiators for adults. Compassion mingles with shame at the ignorance, ineptitude, and identifying accent of the parents who bemoan the increasing impoverishment of family discourse in the mother tongue over the years and the second generation's dismissal of familial custom as eccentric or foreign (often, recouped by the third). As an elderly matriarch, today, more than five decades after migrating to England, I still sometimes grapple with bitter-sweet intricacies of cultural difference, including the lifestyle weirdness of my children and grandchildren, some of whom have themselves migrated elsewhere.

But as ever, reciprocal understanding arises in meaning-making-dialogues to bridge our gaps.

Notes

1 ALSPAC, a longitudinal study of over 10,000 women examined antenatal disturbance separately from postnatal. It found that *severe anxiety* in late pregnancy posed an independent risk associated with behavioural/emotional problems in the school-aged offspring. Maternal "stress" and its concomitant high cortisol levels may be transmitted to the foetus hormonally, producing a hyper-reactive baby, in addition to effects on the gestating foetus of alcohol, nicotine, and opiates imbibed by the anxious mother (see Monk et al., 2020).

2 There are few robust prevalence studies in low and middle income (LMI) societies. A Nuffield meta-analysis of 45 existing studies found that not a single study was conducted in a low-income setting. In other settings, refugee and asylum-seeking women were under-represented; only two intervention studies were identified. A WHO meta-analysis of the sparse data available (from only 8% of LMI societies) suggests that the prevalence of common perinatal mental disorders in low-income countries is *threefold*. One in four women in South Asian countries and up to one in three in South Africa is likely to experience clinical depression after childbirth (due to lack of access to health care; unplanned pregnancy; and poor practical, emotional, and social support for mothers), especially from intimate partners, with low levels of education and high levels of financial insecurity and familial and community violence (Fisher et al., 2012). Even in higher-income societies, up to half of mothers (and a quarter of engaged fathers) experience milder forms of emotional disorders during pregnancy or within the first two years after having a baby. Low social support intensifies adverse factors (eg, poverty, extreme stress, domestic violence, and migration due to natural disasters and conflict situations), increasing the risk for specific disorders. And in pockets of extreme social adversity in high-income societies, rates of clinical depression can range between 32% and 47% during pregnancy and between 16% and 35% during the postnatal period (Tsai & Tomlinson, 2012).

3 Child migrants are especially susceptible to the long-term adverse impact of conflict and displacement. Many witness or experience brutal violence and risk abuse, neglect, exploitation, sex trafficking, or military recruitment. *Medicine*

Sans Frontiers notes an increase in self-harming among children in the detention centre in Lesbos, with self-slashing, headbanging and attendant sleep and eating disorders. Worldwide, there is an urgent need to prioritise the UN 2030 Sustainable Development Goals by investing in young children and their caregivers, especially in refugee settings.

4 Mother-infant dyads with a "traumatic attachment" display acute hyper-responsiveness to each other as a potential threat. Neuroscience research has shown that adrenergic reactions to fear are innate and produced parasympathetically, even in babies. When "flight" or "fight" responses are perceived to increase rather than reduce danger, "freezing" (behaving as if dead) sets in both to confuse predators and to allow pain to be experienced without it being consciously registered (Moore, 2020).

5 Organisations (some of which I was a founding member back in the late 1970s or 1980s) arose to promote scientific perinatal and neonatal research, education, and clinical work through interdisciplinary cooperation. For instance, in the UK, we got the *Royal Society of Medicine* to agree to initiate a subsection on "Maternity and the Newborn" with a multidisciplinary membership of perinatal psychiatrists, psychologists, paediatricians, obstetricians, general practitioners, scientists, academics, midwives, early-childhood nurses, therapists, occupational therapists, community psychiatric nurses, social workers, community nurses, health visitors, and other health professionals. Similarly, the *Marce Society* also came into being in the UK in 1980, to focus specifically on puerperal depression. Today it has become a large international organisation holding regional and biennial congresses to pool scientific knowledge. The *World Association of Infant Mental Health* (WAIMH, founded in the USA, also in 1980) promotes the mental well-being and healthy development of infants through worldwide affiliate associations, with conferences and publications devoted to the study of mental, emotional, and social development during infancy and psychopathological outcomes. *COWAP*, the International Psychoanalytical Association's committee on Women and Psychoanalysis (which I founded in 1998) is now a worldwide organisation with local study groups and international congresses to tease out enigmatic fantasies and unconscious beliefs about the difference between the sexes that underpin the very real and persistent economic, educational, and status gender gap. On a practical level, the Global Alliance for Maternal Mental Health (GAMMH), a coalition of international organisations committed to improving the mental health and well-being of women and their children in pregnancy and the first postnatal year (the *"perinatal period"*) throughout the world, especially under adverse conditions in communities with scarce medical facilities, substandard housing, and few basic services. In the UK, pre- and post-registration training now exists in order to strengthen the understanding and skills of practitioners (www.gov.uk/government/publications/national-perinatal-mental-health-project-report).

6 For instance, the Perinatal Mental Health Project (PMHP) model (https://pmhp.za.org/) includes the provision of screening and counselling for common mental health conditions, integrated into routine maternity care. Concurrent screening for psychosocial risk factors enables the identification of vulnerable groups, such as displaced, migrant, and refugee women. Between the project's inception in September 2002 to end of 2018, 38,991 pregnant women were screened in townships around Cape Town; 6,843 received counselling (19,906 individual sessions). Even after a brief intervention of one to three sessions, 60% of pregnant women reported "much improved" or "complete resolution" of problems relating to primary support, social environment, and lifestyle transition. (Also see Field et al., 2014.)

7 Charlotte Mande Ilunga, a highly experienced counsellor in the PMHP project (above) who has worked in five languages with hundreds of migrants from all

over the continent (ranging from Guinea Bissau in the West to Somalia in the East, and from Algeria in the North to Botswana in the South), spoke to me about cultural and linguistic misunderstanding, which can lead to anxiety, even panic disorder. She shared an anecdote of a couple of political refugees who spoke no English. When the wife defaulted her antenatal appointment as she had a conflicting appointment at the Home Affairs Office, she was handed a card with a date for ANC (Antenatal Clinic). In the absence of an explanation they became alarmed, thinking that they were being sent to attend a political gathering of the ANC. Another point she made was about mothers who struggle a lot with the separation from their newborn, especially when they don't understand why the child is kept in the nursery or in the ICU. "They claim that nursing mothers are like mammals and if separated with their infants it affects the early bonding and connection. They may reject each other. Rooming-in allows the touch, talk, smell and seeing. These things are crucial for the mother-child relationship. Similarly, for some women, the first bathing of the infant is a sacred passage from the amniotic liquid to the natural water. When it is not done, the child is considered unclean until it is done. And when it is done by a stranger, the mother feels cheated in her role as a mother. They feel like the attention is only given to their children and their feelings are not attended. They ask for empathy and not a judgmental attitude filled with prejudice." She adds that even family planning can feel imposed and "counselling in the language a woman understands and expresses freely is a key to an effective therapeutic session."

References

Arendt, H. (1998). *The human condition*. Chicago: The University of Chicago Press.

Bain, K., Landman, M., Frost, K., Raphael-Leff, J., & Baradon, T. (2019). Lay counselors: Thoughts on the crossing of ecological frameworks and the use of lay counselors in the scale up of early infant mental health interventions. *Infant Mental Health Journal*, 1–15. https://doi.org/10.1002/21814.

Bucci, W. (1997). Symptoms and symbols: A multiple code theory of somatization. *Psychoanalytic Inquiry*, *17*, 151–172.

Field, S., Baron, E., Meintjes, I, van Heyningen, T., & Honikman, S. (2014). Maternal mental health care: Refining the components in a South African setting, Chapter 19. In Samuel O. Okpaku (Ed.), *Essentials of global mental health*. Cambridge: Cambridge University Press.

Fisher, J., Mello, C. De, Patel, V., Rahman, A., Tran, T., & Holmes, W. (2012 [2011, November]). Prevalence and determinants of common perinatal mental disorders in women in low- and lower-middle-income countries: A systematic review. *Bulletin of the World Health Organization*, *90*, 139–149.

Monk C., Foss, S., Desaï, P., & Glover, V. (2020). Fetal exposure to mother's distress: New frontiers in research and useful knowledge for daily clinical practice, Chapter 2. In Rosa Maria Quatraro & Pietro Grussu (Eds.), *Handbook of perinatal clinical psychology, from theory to practice* (pp. 26–42). New York and London: Routledge.

Moore, M. S. (2022). Importance of attachment in the presence of a perceived threat. In Valerie Sinason & Renee Potgieter Marks (Eds.), *Treating children with dissociative disorders: Attachment, trauma, theory and practice* (pp. 27–33). London & New York: Routledge.

Morgan, C., & Hutchinson, G. (2010) The social determinants of psychosis in migrant and ethnic minority populations: A public health tragedy. *Psychological Medicine*, *40*(5), 705–709.

Raphael-Leff, J. (2012). *Working with teenage parents: Handbook of theory & practice.* London: Anna Freud Centre.

Raphael-Leff, J. (2017). *Dark side of the womb – pregnancy, parenting and persecutory anxieties.* London: Anna Freud Centre.

Tsai, A. C., & Tomlinson, M. (2012). Mental health spillovers and the millennium development goals: The case of perinatal depression in Khayelitsha, South Africa. *Journal of Global Health, 2*(1), 1–7.

5 Psicólogos Contigo

Working with displaced inhabitants because of a natural disaster

Johanna Mendoza Talledo

> The setting, the frame and all the techniques [that we know inside private practice] could not be replicated here. We only had left "heroic creation."[1] The only thing we had to look for was a shade and two chairs . . ., that was all. . . . [And at the end] the therapeutic dialogue became a bond.
>
> (Member of the White Beard team)

Perú is a country with profound deficiencies in the essential aspects of life. A clear example is the inefficient organisation of the state[2] that expresses itself in the precariousness of our public health system, in a lack of quality education for the majority of the population, as well as in a poor infrastructure. Therefore, any climatic phenomenon or natural disaster can turn into a human catastrophe. Likewise, the neoliberal economic characteristics and social structures that generate racism and discrimination allow us to distinguish processes of marginalisation, exclusion, and extreme poverty of a wide sector of the population, which facilitates the emergence of social catastrophes. Bleichmar (2002) described "surplus discomfort" to refer not only to the discomfort in the culture due to the renunciation of the drives, but also to the one that surpasses us and leads us to abandon the illusion of a full life.

Because of the rains and landslides caused by the phenomenon of the Niño Costero in 2017, the Peruvian Society of Psychoanalysis (SPP) considered it necessary to intervene through a volunteer programme. It assisted the affected population by attending to the psychological effects caused by this climatic emergency that destroyed homes and villages in Perú.

Even though, approximately since the last 40 years, some of the members of the institution have worked with the community in different ways, they have always done it individually or as part of other institutions or projects. For the first time in our institutional history, the SPP began a community policy that allowed joining efforts to

> [c]onsolidate lines of work based on the experience acquired, create an awareness of community work and develop a responsiveness to

DOI: 10.4324/9781003203223-7

national problems. . . . Community work involves the analysts in their own reality, touching them, placing them in the place of helplessness and impotence, for what they require containment and the indispensable institutional support.

(Costa, 2020)

Psicólogos Contigo

In 2017 a wide summons was made to the psychoanalytic-oriented institutions in order to carry out a single and concerted action. In this opportunity, seven institutions responded: they started doing research and sharing technical tools and innovative methodologies, which enhanced the knowledge and experiences of each institution and offered our services as mental health professionals. More than 180 volunteers, between psychology students in their last year, psychotherapists, psychoanalysts, and psychoanalysts-in-training, carried out the interventions. Senior members of the SPP carried out the supervisory work. For the first time, there also was coordination with state institutions (Ministry of Health, Ministry of Education, and Ministry of Women and Vulnerable Populations), which gave a greater capacity for advocacy and presence in the community.

The group that was formed as a result of this summons was called *Psicólogos Contigo* and at the moment consists of the Intercambio Institute, the Vinculare Center, the Psychoanalytic Psychotherapy for Adults Association, the Peruvian Psychoanalytic Psychotherapy of Children and Adolescents Association (APPPNA), the Peruvian Society of Couple and Family Psychoanalytic Psychotherapy, the Expressive Arts Therapies Center (TAE), and the Peruvian Society of Psychoanalysis (SPP).

The initiative of the SPP in the creation and consolidation of the project gives it visibility not only among psychoanalytic institutions, but also in the academic world and in society as a whole. The formation of a group of institutions enhances the capacities for action, allowing the SPP to lead a work movement to attend to the urgent needs of the population (Costa, 2020).

Up to 2019, *Psicólogos Contigo* has generated four projects:

1   Assistance in the field (2017–2018): volunteers were trained, and four groups were formed to assist areas around Lima in a state of emergency: Barba Blanca, Cajamarquilla, and Ñaña. The work was with adults, adolescents, and children.

2   The application of the notebook *My History about the Landslides and Floods in Perú* El Niño Costero 2017–2018 (Cajamarquilla). This notebook was designed to promote elaboration processes of the disruptive impact in children between 7 and 12 years old, and it was given to 1,825 girls and boys. It was developed based on a methodological

model designed by the Mercy Corps after the terrorist attacks to the Twin Towers in 2001.

3   Prevention against violence of girls and boys at the Fe y Alegría School in Pamplona Alta (2019) where attention strategies and group techniques were developed. Three hundred families were assisted.
4   Together with the Ministry of Education, a project on prevention of violence against girls and boys at school was proposed (2019). The pilot plan developed had five components but has been put on hold due to the pandemic, with the hope of being resumed in the near future.

In 2019, the project *Psicólogos Contigo* received the first prize for best project of "IPA in the Community" and the "Presidency Award."

During the pandemic, the Peruvian Society of Psychoanalysis continued its committed work with the community: (1) the preparation of *Informative Primers*[3] was carried out; (2) an *Emotional Support Line*[4] was created; (3) group work called *Listening Time*[5] was carried out, and (4) a project is currently being developed with the *MINSA*[6] (Ministry of Health).

Barba Blanca: the volunteers as a transformational object

Next, I will present an analysis of the material that appears in a video produced by the Barba Blanca team between 2018 and 2019. Taking the aforementioned eight-minute video[7] as a starting point, I will use the dialogues of the participants to offer some psychoanalytic afterthoughts on the experience, the psychoanalytic technique used, and on the feminine aspects of work, the subject of the IPA congress in London in 2019.

Transcript of the video dialogues

Villager of Barba Blanca speaks in voice over:

The landslide has ruined the whole town.
Around 50 families used to live here.
It is uncommunicated.
There is no vehicular access.
All this was Barba Blanca.

In March 2017, El Niño damaged the town of Barba Blanca, Huarochirí, in the highlands of Lima, Perú. The support between the neighbours prevented human losses and facilitated people's migration towards higher and safer areas. However, the landslide buried almost every house and crop field.

SILVANA GAZZO: We arrived at Barba Blanca aiming to help but without knowing how, or when, or anything! We only had a question mark in our minds. As we arrived, the truth is that reality is always worse than fiction, because we found pain, we found rupture . . . rupture among many things. Among the villagers, the geographical displacement of their homes meant that, in some cases, family members were also separated. There were parents who slept in a tent and their children in a temporary shelter. These were small, so the families had to split up, which might seem not important, but it is essential, because the children started having fears. The sounds, any rain alert meant the possibility of living this again.

LILIAN FERREYROS: The Peruvian Psychoanalytic Society created an organisation called *Psychologist with You*, whose members responded to the disaster by assisting the population not in the material reconstruction, but in the reconstruction of their internal world.

SG: As we arrived, we met an organisation's female leader who told us about the population. We realised we could work with children, adolescents, and adults.

LF: It was a challenge for us, who were used to work within private practice, to take psychoanalysis outside the consulting room. What were we going to find? How were we going to work? Would it be only listening, and holding? Were we going to focus on the landslide experience, the losses? Somehow, we improvised "on the go" a way of working with our tools.

SG: The way we intervened ended up being what we've called therapeutic dialogues, because the setting, the frame, and all the traditional techniques could not be replicated here. It was a heroic creation! We had to figure out how to do it, how? The only thing we had to find was a shade and two chairs. What was the approach? Honestly, it was very easy because these people were full of so much pain that we only had to listen. At the beginning, it was only listening, and then it became a dialogue, given that we could not work in depth, it ended up being a human conversation about the pain they felt. That was the only thing we could do.

LF: With the children, we worked with play boxes, and we realised that every child re-signified the landslide in his or her own way. The first day, we noticed that many of the girls introduced themselves with different names as if they were their own. "Elsa," said two of them. We realised those were not their names. Who was Elsa? Gradually, we realised Elsa was a Walt Disney character who had the power of transforming things into ice and snow, especially when she was furious or stressed. This figure was interesting: a girl with the power of destruction, like the landslide, but who in peaceful times was a princess, happy and beautiful. They built erupting volcanoes, they played war; there is some parricide: sometimes they played frying their fathers. Every three Sundays, we visit them. These children waited for us with a need to play and express themselves.

SG: A bond was established. . . . [T]he therapeutic dialogue managed to become a bond.

Dialogue analysis

The video begins with the voiceover of a villager of Barba Blanca who describes the misfortune that occurred. I will highlight three points:

(1) The landslide and the floods **swept** the whole town.
(2) Barba Blanca **has no communication**.
(3) **There is no access**.

This was the unfathomable way of expressing the impact suffered by the force of nature (water and floods), by the great material losses (houses, crops, even animals), and fundamentally, by the disruptive experience in the psyche of the inhabitants. The first words we heard in the video allowed us to represent their experience: swept up, isolated, and without access to their ego and emotional resources.

Disruptive events have the capacity to break into the psyche and produce reactions that alter the capacity for integration and elaboration (Benyakar, 2003). The approach to this type of event, in this case rains and landslides of neighbouring hills, has the particularity of having an impact not only on the affected population but also on the therapists who participate "in the reconstruction of the internal world." The experiences and the destruction suffered by the population affected the Barba Blanca team.

At the beginning of the video, Silvana G. enunciates the disruptiveness in the team. She expresses the horror the volunteers met: "[T]he truth," she says, "is that reality is always worse than fiction, because we find pain, we find rupture . . . rupture of a lot of things." She talks about separations, between parents and children, between siblings; about losses, threats, and the fears the children felt. Silvana G. also states that they did not count with the known technical instruments, that all kinds of "usual frame" disappeared and that they only had "a question mark in their minds." Lilian F. would add: "It was a challenge for us . . . to take the psychoanalysis out of the private practice, what were we going to find, how were we going to work?"

The disruptive aspect of the reality, which unexpectedly and surprisingly brought destruction and damage to the inhabitants of Barba Blanca, produced reactions that altered the capacity for integration and elaboration of the Barba Blanca team. The video shows a village half buried between mud and stones (external world) and, in correspondence, were the minds of the volunteers . . . swept away, deinstrumentalised with experiences of collapse, with some split mind aspects? Were they disorganised by the impact of the pain and the death anguish they saw? In this type of experience, we as analysts have to add an extra effort to elaborate the exposure to the destabilising impact of the disruptive situation (Benyakar, 2003).

After this first moment, the observation and the listening of the volunteers focused on what had not been destroyed. They aimed to link with the community "organisation," so they looked for the town's leader, a woman who at that time was in charge of organising the meals, and spoke with her to get to know what the population was like. This is precisely the opposite of "remaining uncommunicated." This is meeting the "organisation," the resources. We witnessed the search for connection, for bonding, for identifying the organised and creative aspects that existed both in the community's inhabitants and in their own minds.

The team realised that there had not been human losses. The video shows us, over time the residents and volunteers playing soccer, painting, playing with play boxes, having "therapeutic dialogues" inside a van, sitting under a shade in some corner of the town. You cannot "trace or copy" the conditions of a private practice; the only option left is to perform a "heroic creation" – that is, a creation with great effort and improvising solutions.

They were able to return to what Lilian had pointed out: *the objective was to assist the population in the reconstruction of their internal world.* The volunteers felt again that *"with their tools"* they could let themselves go out to meet the spontaneous gesture. It would be more accurate to say the gesture of pain, of anger, but also of hope, to continue listening analytically, held in their internal frame, a cardinal concept in contemporary psychoanalytic thinking. An example of this is when Lilian F. can understand who Elsa is, this Disney character, and can attribute an analytical sense to her.

New spaces were constructed that facilitated access roads for the establishment of a co-metabolising bond and acting as a structuring object and as a transformational object (Benyakar, 2003). Because of this, we understand how, at the end of the video, Silvana G. could manage to part by saying: "[T]he therapeutic dialogue managed to become a bond."

The feminine at work with the community

If we could rewind what was seen in the video or what we just read in the *transcript of the video dialogues*, we could identify expressions and concepts associated with the feminine. There are many possible ways of thinking about the feminine. In this paper I will pick up only two: Bion's concept of daydream or *reverie* (1962) that indicates the state of receptivity of the mother to receive, digest, and give meaning to the feelings and anguish of the infant – namely, the mother as a metabolising agent of the beta elements, converting them into alpha ones. Would Bion be allowing us to infer that the *reverie*, besides an experience of necessary maternal care for the psychic survival of the baby, is a feminine psychic attribute?

A second topic: there are experiences that favour deep regressions and may force us to re-experience what it is to feel helpless, needy, frustrated, furious, tormented, abandoned (Raphael-Leff, 1988) and that reveal fragile and vulnerable states and the manifestation of primitive aspects (Kristeva, 1980, 1988). These are statements from Julia Kristeva and Joan Raphael-Leff about the representations of the emotional states of women in their experiences of pregnancy, childbirth, and initial care of their baby, making visible those first sensations or nameless registries. All of us have recorded these experiences because we all are children of someone.

In the work with the population exposed to disruptive events, it is necessary that volunteers can offer, not exclusively, of course, but in an indispensable way, their capacity for *reverie* and maternal function, despite the feelings of fragility and vulnerability in which they find themselves due to the exposure to pain and loss experiences of the villagers. Knowing their work with detail provides us with information, to have support and accompaniment criteria in this approach and to cooperate in the generation of the co-metaboliser bond between the community and the voluntary analysts and between the latter and their colleagues and the institution.

Cesar Vallejo (1987), a Peruvian poet considered by some as "the greatest poet of the twentieth century," said that *"every great act or voice comes from the people and goes to the people,"* highlighting that all human creation is born from the culture where we are all rooted, all without exception. I would like to transfer this verse to the field of knowledge: any discipline, psychoanalysis in our case, was a brilliant act produced in the 20th century. It is our commitment to continuously re-create it in dialogue with the culture from which it emerges and where it belongs.

Notes

1 The complete sentence "neither tracing nor copy but heroic creation" belongs to José Carlos Mariátegui, Peruvian writer, journalist, and politician, published in the *Amauta Journal*, no. 17, in September 1928. Natalia Majluf, curator of the *Amauta Exhibition* (2019), exhibited at the Lima Art Museum (MALI), pointed out that this was a deep cultural and political project of Mariátegui, who proposed to think the reality of Perú as complex at the same time as unique – therefore "neither tracing nor copying" of other realities. The word "heroic" is understood as the accomplishment of a great feat, as creating with great effort, many times from nothing, and inventing solutions.
2 That became evident in the pandemic generated by COVID-19, which claimed 180,000 lives till May 2021.
3 One booklet for the general public, another one for first-line personnel (health workers, doctors, firefighters, supply managers), a third one for the police forces and the armed forces, a fourth booklet for the elderly and the last one about duelling (Costa, 2020).
4 About 5,000 telephone calls were answered to contain anxiety and validate feelings of sadness, anger, depression, and anxiety as natural emotions (Costa, 2020).
5 Listening and containment of the experiences in their daily work with COVID-19, strengthening emotional and professional resources, advocating for bonding and group aspects to strengthen the task. It was carried out virtually with mixed teams of professionals who worked on the front line: prosecutors, police,

members of mental health centres, social workers, and lawyers in Loreto and Cuzco (Costa, 2020).

6 Contact was established with the Mental Health Area of the Ministry of Health to work with the Community Mental Health Centers. Currently, work with more than 20 CSMCs has been registered.

7 You can access the video "Secuelas del Niño Costero en Barba Blanca 2017" at https://youtu.be/aycdEiYIQi4

References

Benyakar, M. (2003). *Lo disruptivo. Amenazas individuales y colectivas: el psiquismo entre guerras, terrorismos y catastrofes sociales.* Buenos Aires: Editorial Biblos.

Bion, W. R. (1962). The psyco-analytic study of thinking. *International Journal of Psychoanalysis, 43.*

Bleichmar, S. (2002). *Dolor país.* Buenos Aires: Libros del Zorzal.

Costa, M. P. (2020). *Psicologos Contigo. Congreso online de la API en la Comunidad. Psicoanálisis mas allá del diván.* Webinar. Retrieved from https://youtube.be/-k2t3oYeYTg.

Kristeva, J. (1980). *Desire in language.* Nueva York: Columbia Press.

Kristeva, J. (1988). *Los poderes de la perversión.* Buenos Aires: Siglo XXl.

Raphael-Leff, J. (1988). El lugar de las cosas Salvajes. En *Mujeres por Mujeres.* Lima: Biblioteca Peruana de Psicoanálisis.

Vallejo, C. (1987). *España, aparta de mí este caliz.* Madrid: Editorial Castalia.

6 From a trench in the war against children

Gilbert Kliman

A number of colleagues have asked me how a psychoanalyst, such as I, became involved in community activities, including the pursuit of social justice through psychoanalytically informed expert witness services. I am glad to provide some autobiographical information, since it may cast some light on how others could be involved. My autobiography includes transgenerational influences, parts of which I will briefly sketch.

Holocaust and pogrom deaths were numerous among the close relatives of both my maternal and paternal grandparents. A genetic disorder called Lynch Syndrome led to 15 deaths of paternal family members before and while I was a child. It ultimately invaded my father, two of my sons, and myself with various potentially or actually deadly carcinomas. Some are plaguing me to this day. My childhood did not include a conscious understanding of these influences. Instead, when I had numerous surgeries at ages two, three, and four, I felt the anxieties of my parents, grandparents, aunts, and uncles that I – at that time the only child and only grandchild – might not survive. My dearest and most caregiving grandmother fell silent for three months in my early childhood upon learning by mail of her Odessa family's obliteration in a pogrom. The surrounding fearful protectiveness caused a counterphobic and constructively independent trend which has pervaded my entire life. A demand to be free of the structures and fears of my personal and my familial past has motivated much of my relationship to psychoanalysis. Early on, I became intellectually and physically independent and took much pleasure in archaeologic and aviation adventures beyond the comfort and ken of my relatives.

In my teens, I was a leader of civil rights activities. I defied the Ku Klux Klan at the Mason Dixon line, integrating a college dormitory, nearby restaurants and an interstate bus long before Rosa Parks. As a counterphobic youth during a summer, I earned well by mining lead and zinc 900 feet underground, beneath a river in Idaho, using dynamite skilfully. I became a pilot in my early twenties and continued to use the aviation skill to go back and forth to the Mexican Border for a project about which I will summarise shortly below. Trained at a constraining psychoanalytic institute, I took childlike joy in going beyond the bounds of office practice, setting

DOI: 10.4324/9781003203223-8

up research projects, loss and trauma–focused major clinics and applications of child analysis, which were at the time quite unusual.

The particular focus of this chapter represents an epiphany based upon decades of psychoanalytic experience with traumatised persons, combined with my knowledge of expert psychoanalytic testimony. That testimony usually concerns the pursuit of compensation for psychological damages inflicted upon children within various institutional settings. It was in May 2018 while at a conference of the American Psychoanalytic Association that I had the beginnings of the epiphany. I was in my hotel room thinking of retiring from my labours as I neared 90 years of age. Meanwhile my wife, Harriet Wolfe, was busy being president of an organisation which then seemed focused upon its survival as a guild, an association which seemed to be cutting itself off from the terrible outside world in which traumas were being inflicted by our own government upon helpless people. Within the halls of the conference hotel there was much turmoil about the psychoanalytic method. Was method A better than psychoanalytic method B? Was three times a week or five times a week the holy grail? Some serious practitioners seemed to damn those who did not practice according to seemingly sacred and apparently tribal precepts of one or another tribe of psychoanalysts.

At that very time I was hearing on radio and television and Google news that US attorney general Jeff Sessions and President Donald Trump were criminalising the previous misdemeanour of seeking asylum through informal means rather than coming to immigration stations. As a deterrent, a barbaric practice was being enacted in the name of our government supposedly protecting our nation from another tribal threat. That imagined threat was an invasion, an imagined wave of rapists, criminals, and other bad people from a supposedly undesirable and different tribe. As a matter of policy, as had been done by our government to Native Americans and African American slaves, children were being separated from their parents. Some were caged and put into so-called concrete cells, violating international standards of humane treatment of refugees. I thought to myself how ironic that psychoanalysts were meeting in this hotel to deal with patients who were often the victims of various childhood traumas, while we were doing nothing much to prevent the large-scale infliction of known traumatic harms. The harms were inflicted under the banner of our own taxpayer-supported immigration authorities. Private jails contracted with our taxpayers supported the government in mistreating asylum seekers.

It occurred to me that many other psychoanalysts might view the separations as I did. Perhaps they would be sufficiently frustrated with working on the results of trauma when they might reach out and prevent traumas. Thus, while still at the meeting, I decided not to retire. Instead, I resumed my adolescent civil rights activist mode. In that frame of mind, I sent out a large number of emails to colleagues requesting that they join me under the umbrella of the Children's Psychological Health Center, a non-profit agency I direct. They could volunteer to perform forensic evaluations on asylum seekers, getting some training and supervision from me. It was my theory that the asylum seekers were deliberately not being listened to by immigration authorities and that psychoanalytic ears would listen well. Potentially, psychoanalysts could be trained to record their hearing and provide expert reports about the overlooked or deliberately unheard reasons for asylum seekers to seek a haven in the United States. In this effort, I was rewarded with an almost immediate response by about 115 colleagues who were willing to provide their services, pro bono, to asylum seekers. This was a first step.

It was not sufficient that I offered our agency's now expanded services to many attorneys and organisations dealing with asylum seekers. For weeks and months I got no takers of our collective willingness. It was fortunate that my wife, Harriet Wolfe, needed occasional relief from her duties in the guild. She sometimes sought it with a group of women called the "Cookettes," who practiced teaching each other culinary arts in their homes. Harriet felt my distress and expressed from time to time my frustration with the lack of attorneys using my services which had been so valuable to non-asylum-seekers. One of the Cookettes was an immigration attorney who had contributed services to asylum seekers. She gave my name to RAICES, a non-profit organisation working at the Texas Mexico border with asylum seekers. Finally, through this very informal personal connection, I was invited to visit child and parent refugees jailed in private profitable jails in Dilley, Texas, and later to Karnes, Texas.

It was clear to me and my team that the attorneys involved in most of the cases had no experience with how powerful a psychological damage suit can be against an institution. They, in fact, would not listen to me on the subject. They literally would not correspond with me on the subject. However, my nickname being "persistence," I tried to live up to my nominal identity. That is when among over 50 asylum seekers my team had evaluated, I encountered a set of 13 fathers and their 13 sons who had been twice separated from each other. The second separation was apparently done with malicious forethought, without due process, and despite copious warnings against the harm which would likely be done. I realised there was probably an incontrovertible set of facts which could be introduced in court as the basis for a psychological damage suit.

I then cultivated the friendship of Curtis Doebbler, an attorney working in Texas with RAICES. He had also worked with Nelson Mandela. I told him of my civil rights interests and then decades of cumulatively reaching multibillion-dollar awards and settlements on behalf of children and other traumatises plaintiffs in "civilian" cases. He listened carefully and decided to proceed. He obtained the help of a law firm, Arendt Fox, which provided experienced litigators who knew about civil suits, not just about asylum-seeking suits.

While we were preparing the litigation for psychological damages, it seemed to me that Curtis became inspired, and his whole organisation took on a creative task, for which I take no credit. They raised millions of dollars to provide bail for hundreds of asylum seekers who were in jails awaiting their delayed due process. This took the private jails and associated federal authorities by surprise, and hundreds of jailed asylum seekers were suddenly released.

A video of a child being interviewed by me was shown to the United Nations and persuaded the viewers that the United States had indeed violated international law in the treatment of these fathers and sons. The boy described the removal of his father by armed guards, his own removal to a medical facility; he remembered being told falsely that he would never see his father again and that his father was in jail for being a terrorist. According to the boy's vivid account, there was a pastor who came to the medical facility to which the terror-stricken boy was removed. The pastor prayed for the fathers and sons. A woman psychologist came to treat them. Medications were offered, and guards laughed mockingly at the crying children. The fathers had meanwhile been overnight in distant solitary isolation cells, shackled, dehydrated, and accused of terrorism, with no charges brought. They were returned the next day. Some of the fathers and sons were clearly no longer the same, suffering from posttraumatic damages which the suit will articulate.

The complaint against the private jail includes the following language, much of it inspired by my views and advice:

Complaint

COME NOW, Plaintiffs, by and through their attorneys of record, and for their Complaint against Defendant The GEO Group, Inc. ("GEO"), state:

General allegations

1   Plaintiffs are thirteen asylum-seeking children and their thirteen asylum-seeking FATHERS who fled persecution and violence threatening their well-being or lives in their home countries to seek protection in the United States. Pursuant to the federal government's "zero tolerance policy," Plaintiff FATHERS were forcibly separated from their respective sons after they entered the United States. In implementing such policy the federal government relied on companies, such as Defendant The GEO Group, Inc. ("GEO"), to manage and operate detention centers where Plaintiffs would be held indefinitely pending resolution of their claims for protection. Plaintiffs' claims arise from GEO's intentional misconduct and mistreatment of them while GEO detained them at the Karnes County Residential Center (the "Karnes Detention Center") in Karnes City, Texas, and/or the

South Texas Detention Complex (the "Pearsall Detention Center") in Pearsall, Texas.

2   On June 26, 2018, the United States District Court for the Southern District of California issued a nationwide preliminary injunction (the "Preliminary Injunction") prohibiting the Immigration and Customs Enforcement ("ICE"), the Department of Homeland Security ("DHS"), United States Customs and Border Patrol ("CBP"), their officers and agents, and those participating with them from detaining those parent class members in "[Department of Homeland Security] custody without and apart from their minor children." *Ms. L v. I.C.E., et al.*[1] That court found that family separation severely harms children and parents alike.[2] Pursuant to the Preliminary Injunction, parent class members were to be reunited with their minor children who were (i) under the age of five within fourteen (14) days, and (ii) age five (5) and above within thirty (30) days.[3] Plaintiffs in this case, all of whom were covered by the Preliminary Injunction, were reunited and subsequently detained at the Karnes Detention Center.

3   Upon information and belief, with no prior notice, in direct violation of the Preliminary Injunction and with callous indifference toward Plaintiffs' rights, on August 15, 2018, GEO re-separated Plaintiff children from their Plaintiff FATHERS without a lawful justification (the "08/15/2018 Re-separation"), in violation of the court-ordered reunification, and in violation of the constitutional rights of the FATHERS and their children. GEO directed, arranged, participated, and/or permitted scores of armed men to forcibly apprehend Plaintiff FATHERS, handcuff them, and remove them from the Karnes Detention Center by using excessive force and carrying gear including bulletproof vests, shields, kneepads, boots, helmets, tear gas equipment, and guns. When removing the FATHERS, officers pointed their rifles and pistols at them and/or made statements unnecessarily causing them to fear for their lives. GEO then removed the FATHERS without their children from the Karnes Detention Center, loaded them onto a bus, and transported them with all of their belongings to the Pearsall Detention Center, nearly two hours away. GEO refused to inform the FATHERS where they were being taken, why GEO was again separating them from their children, whether the children would remain at the Karnes Detention Center or anywhere in the United States, whether their children were safe, and who would care for them. GEO's staff also told the FATHERS that they would be deported without their children, that their children would be adopted by families living in the United States, and that they would never again see their children.

4   Upon information and belief, Plaintiff FATHERS cried while GEO removed the FATHERS with all their belongings from the Karnes Detention Center and transferred them to the Pearsall Detention

Center. GEO's actions caused the FATHERS to suffer great mental distress, trauma, and anguish. Once they arrived at the Pearsall Detention Center GEO removed the FATHERS from the bus; formally processed them through intake procedures at the Pearsall Detention Center; and gave the FATHERS handbooks and rules for the Pearsall Detention Center, uniforms, and identification bracelets. GEO's actions caused the FATHERS to reasonably believe that they would be indefinitely detained there alone and that they would never see their children again.

5   Upon information and belief, while GEO removed Plaintiff FATHERS from the Karnes Detention Center, GEO told Plaintiff children (who were as young as six years old) that they were going to be separated again from their FATHERS permanently. GEO told the Plaintiff children that their Plaintiff FATHERS would never return to the Karnes Detention Center and mocked the Plaintiff children by saying, among other things, "Don't worry, your fathers are in jail."

6   Upon information and belief, for an unjust number of hours following the 08/15/2018 Re-separation, Plaintiff children had no idea where their FATHERS were, Plaintiff FATHERS had no idea where their children were, and GEO intentionally refused to respond to Plaintiffs' inquiries about the location, safety, and well-being of their loved ones. In fact, GEO laughed at and ridiculed both the FATHERS and the children, making fun of their dire circumstances and exacerbating the extreme distress caused by the re-separation from their loved ones. GEO's deliberate actions traumatized Plaintiff FATHERS and children and intentionally subjected them to severe and continuing emotional distress, psychological trauma, and mental anguish. GEO's actions also violated Plaintiff FATHERS' statutory rights under Texas law to possession of and access to their children.

The above matter is pending, and I hope to testify, or that the matter will "settle" with financial compensation for the victims, permitting them to rehabilitate.

In conclusion, I want to encourage my fellow psychoanalysts and psychoanalytically oriented psychotherapists to come out of their offices and go into the community. There they will find many ways to multiply the effectiveness of their training and help a larger number of patients than they could treat on a one-to-one basis. I further invite the readers of this volume to study another method with me called Reflective Network Therapy, which multiplies the effectiveness of a child therapist, multiplying the number of preschool age patients she or he can treat. It avoids dropout. It creates a field of analytically workable information within the natural setting of a preschool patient's own classroom. The network consists of an index patient, teachers, parents, and non-patient preschoolers.

The method may be understood as an application of field theory. It allows the in-classroom field to be used as a medium for interpreting transference and a child's historical and current relational conflicts. This occurs while developing mentalising functions within the field of the index patient. Up to 8 or 12 preschool patients may be treated every day by a therapist within a collaborating preschool.

There are videotaped trainings which may permit you to carry out this technique yourselves in preschools near you, creating a ripple of vulnerable children's mental health and recovery in your own communities. It has greater power and public health reach than you could wield by treating preschool patients dyadically.

Our recordings of forensic trainings are also available. The two agencies I direct have websites at www.childrenspsychologicalhealthcenter.org and *www.TheHarlemFamilyInstitute.org*. I am so grateful that my contribution in this volume offers the possibility to relate to many other colleagues who are engaged with traumatised children, adolescents, and adults worldwide.

Notes

1 310 F.Supp.3d 1133, 1149 (S.D.Cal. 2018).
2 *Id.*
3 *Id.* at 1149.

Bibliography

Black, P. H. (2003). The inflammatory response is an integral part of the stress response: Implications for atherosclerosis, insulin resistance, type II diabetes and metabolic syndrome X. *Brain Behav Immun, 17*(5), 350–364. Epub 2003/08/30. pmid:12946657.

Bucci, M., Marques, S. S., Oh, D., & Harris, N. B. (2016). Toxic stress in children and adolescents. *Advances in Pediatrics, 63*(1), 403–428. pmid:27426909

Kliman, G. (1968). *Psychological emergencies of childhood*. New York: Grune and Stratton.

Kliman, G. (2009). Voices for psychologically injured children: Psychoanalytic testimony during civil litigation helps bring social change, settlements, and jury awards. *Psychoanalytic Inquiry, 20*, 6.

Kliman, G. (2011). *Reflective network therapy in the preschool classroom*. Lanham, MD: University Press of America.

Miller, T., Waehrer, G. M., Oh, D. L., Boparai, S. P., Walker, S. O., Marques, S. S., & Harris, N. B. (2020). Adult health burden and costs in California during 2013 associated with prior adverse childhood experiences. *PLoS One, 15*, 1.

7 Suffering from elsewhere

Trauma and its transmission

Debra Gill

Introduction

Psychoanalysis is collectively beginning to examine how human tragedies emerging from legacies of violence, oppression, and environmental disasters impact internal life, shaping the lens of psychic reality. The broader sociopolitical world brings the history of genocide, war, and displacement, as well as racialised and gendered oppression, into the dimensions of the psychoanalytic field. The transmission of intergenerational trauma from the Holocaust has been studied extensively, and in recent decades, the impact of migration, exile, and immigration (Akhtar, 1999) on future generations has become an area of continued research and thought. In the face of the gross racial inequities exposed during COVID-19, psychoanalysis is beginning to confront the dangerous idealisation of whiteness (Suchet, 2007; Moss, 2021), and through that exploration, examine the trauma of racism that has reverberated across generations of African Americans specifically in the United States (Holmes, 2016; Powell, 2018; Stoute, 2017). Globally, the generations closest to genocide, war, exile, and racialised violence are understandably too close to trauma and its aftermath to mentally represent horrific experiences. Next-generation survivors are left to psychically metabolise inherited trauma, and since human violation is perpetuated, many from this new generation will face their own oppression and suffering.

Trauma transmitted from an ancestral past seeks repetition and will find refuge not only within the patient but in the unconscious coupling of the analytic dyad. This chapter will consider how the multifocal lens of the analytic field offers opportunities for a broader frame capable of holding the dimensioned levels of turbulence carried through intergenerational trauma.

Après-Coup of Intergenerational Trauma

Haydee Faimberg's (2005) seminal work on the telescoping of intergenerational trauma offers a psychoanalytic framework for listening and thinking

DOI: 10.4324/9781003203223-9

about the families of those who survived genocide and war. Telescoping is defined as the unconscious transmission of trauma that is temporally displaced through narcissistic identification so that traumatic events from previous generations are carried into the psyches of the present generations. Internalised parents appropriate and intrude on psychic space, impacting the next generation's capacity to achieve psychic separateness. Intergenerational survivors, therefore, live with the remains of all that could not be held in mind by previous generations. Through unconscious identifications, this population suffers disordered attachment (Grand & Salberg, 2017) and structural problems that rely on early defences such as dissociation, somatisation, and destructive action (Apprey, 2017). Unrepresented trauma is transmitted and not mourned.

This chapter will consider the generativity of the field, first as a holding space (Winnicott, 1956), where the analyst can reliably anchor the frame, and second as a field that will allow the matrix of psychic trauma, hidden in transmission, to find expression. In cases of trauma transmission, the field is thought about as an intermediate or transitional space comprising an expanded, intersecting framework. The lived experiences between patient and analyst are unconsciously enacted until the analyst can interpret the field through a new narrative. Traumatic events that are situated in a disavowed past can be recollected as distant and organised facts but are without emotional meaning. The analytic field offers the potential for an emergent narrative that can mobilise stagnant events into the mental arena of thinking.

To advance thinking and re-work psychic events, Faimberg (1996) and others suggest a broader conceptualisation of *Nachträglichkeit*, defined originally by Freud in a letter to Fleiss as occurring "when memory traces acquire new meaning" (Faimberg, 2005). The process of assigning new and reflective meaning to a disavowed traumatic event in the service of bringing about psychic change expands both the definition and function of *Nachträglichkeit*, or from the French, *Après-Coup*. The temporal dimensions of trauma operate unconsciously so that a historical event can be re-experienced in the present and through a different lens can be altered in service of broadening psychic reality. Within the psychoanalytic field, transmitted trauma can acquire retroactive meaning for a next-generation survivor.

The Field as a Dimensioned Analytic Space

According to Katz and Civitarese (2017), a central origin of field theory emerged through the work of Kurt Lewin, a German American Gestalt psychologist who was exiled from his birth origin. He proposed that behaviour is the result of the individual in interaction with a dynamic social environment. In her pioneering and expansive research of the analytic field, Katz emphasises that field theory encompasses a broad spectrum of influence, including Lewin's social psychology and its emphasis on interdependence. She speaks about how social psychology dovetailed with the postmodern trend that centralises the narrative, two-person exchange inherent of the psychoanalytic process. The environmental matrix of conscious and unconscious relating was brought into psychoanalysis through relational theorists in the United States, beginning with Jay Greenberg and Stephen Mitchell in 1983. Through the lens of object relations, the relational theorists grouped together an alternative to drive theory, one that posited relationships as central in theoretical systems (Mitchell et al., 1999). As relational theory expanded, a central tenet of classical theory was called into question – namely, the analyst's realistic capacity for neutrality and objectivity. The endorsement of a two-person psychology rooted in intersubjectivity and involvement with the patient (Renik, 1999) was identified by emerging influencers of an expanding school of psychoanalysis. From the relational perspective, enactment is necessary and central to analysing countertransference. These ideas, all inherent in a two-person psychology contributed to the developing analytic field.

Years prior to relational analysis, and clearly having had an impact on contemporary contributions, South American and European analysts developed the origins of the relational field. The work of Baranger and Baranger (2008), originating in South America 1961, is considered both foundational and expansive in terms of bringing in a wider experience of psychoanalysis technically and theoretically. While Baranger and Baranger (2008) did not emphasise the sociocultural elements of the field, they pioneered the centrality of a bi-personal dimension where the countertransference and transference were considered equally important. While the contributions are of equal importance, in this model the analyst is considered responsible for both shaping and tolerating the uncertainty of treatment.

Martin Silverman (2017) adds to the Barangers' field dimension and the influence of what he calls the "immediate surround," defined by the sociocultural climate and geography: the state, city, or neighbourhood, asking where does the analysis occur, and how does location impact the dyad? Historically, analysis has taken place in the context of war, political division, racialised disparity, and recently, through a pandemic. Analysts who escaped fascism in Europe, and did not emigrate to the United States, were more accepting of the analyst's own cumulative contributions to the field, which, according to Silverman (2017), began with the work of Melanie Klein. In a review of volumes of work on field theory, far and wide, Silverman captures how the originators of theory in South America, who were forced to flee Europe in the 1930s to escape the rise of Nazism, studied psychosis through Klein. After the war, many South Americans studied in London and relied on Klein's expansive theories to reach children and adults in psychotic states. Her expanded theories of early defences like splitting, projective identification, envy, and the death instinct, like Freud's, offer a philosophy of humanity and the challenges to civilisation that encompass love and hate. Klein's expansion of unconscious phantasy includes the presence of an internal object at the beginning of life. Based in the presence of a maternal object, the dyadic world was developed by D. W. Winnicott and Wilfred Bion, both of whom are considered central to laying the groundwork for a two-person analytic model. The Winnicottian theory of the facilitating environment relied on the centrality of the mother and her capacity to facilitate transitional functioning for the infant (Winnicott, 1953). In adulthood, the achievement of transitional capacity leads to a negotiation of internal and external reality – a functional intermediate mental space required to develop separateness, thought, and symbolism.

Bion's theory of the container/contained (1962) centres on the mother/analyst's mental capacity to receive and transform the raw sensations of infantile elements into digestible and dreamable thoughts that can be used by the adult patient to think and expand. In both these models, the analyst, in a two-person experience, shapes the field by relying on the maternal, analytic function of containment. In the post-Bionian field developed by Antonino Ferro and Giuseppe Civitarese, the field is understood experientially within the moment to moment interplay of the analytic couple. (Civaterese and Ferro, 2018) The evolving couple dynamics enables reverie, dreaming and the development of a transformational field, allowing for new narratives and psychic expansion.

The analytic field, when developed into a furtive transitional or intermediate space, allows for the emergence of trauma transmitted from elsewhere. Psychic trauma that reverberates through a time capsule, *après-coup* in the field, offers an opportunity for a revised and fluid meaning of intergenerational experiences that have been frozen and static.

Alexandra Woods (2020) in her article "The Work before Us: Whiteness and the Psychoanalytic Institute" discusses how psychoanalysts who eventually emigrated to the United States, escaping war and Nazi persecution, needed to disavow trauma to fit into American institutes where the analysis of internal forces was elevated above all other factors. Woods notes that trauma from a societal context was considered extra-analytic, and individuals needed to meet criteria for analysability in order to be considered for analysis. Whiteness, while not specified, is implicated. Not until Dorothy Holmes (1992) and Kimberlyn Leary (1997) brought the experience of race in the transference into psychoanalytic discourse was racial difference in the analytic dyad thought about dimensionally. Intergenerational trauma, based in the US history of slavery and segregation, including systemic oppression and violence to African American communities, were not emphasised in psychoanalytic theory or practice. Beverly

Stoute (2017) questions whether unexamined racism in psychoanalysis is indicative of unmetabolised transmission and believes that psychoanalysis can attenuate destructive trends in the profession and the larger socio-political world.

Two composite case studies follow that illustrate how intergenerational trauma is released, *après-coup* through the field, presenting opportunities for an expansion of psychic reality.

Notes from the Field: Two Case Illustrations of Intergenerational Trauma

Underground Whispers, NYC Post 9/11

Ms A. came to treatment when she was in her early forties. During her early latency years her family was forced to flee their country of origin to escape religious and political persecution. Ms A. began therapy with me in NYC, not too long after 9/11. The city, at the time, was on edge after the attack, and in the immediate surround were incidents of brown-skinned people who were profiled as suspected terrorists. It was common for people of colour to be subjected to random searches, particularly in the subway. Living under suspicion was commonplace, and many brown-skinned people affixed small pins of the American Flag on an article of clothing to signify their support for the United States and offset any linkage to the perception of threatening other.

Adding to all the conscious and unconscious complexities of the field include an analytic dyad of different origins, each raised in a different sociocultural world. In the aftermath of 9/11, I, the white analyst, did not suffer othering and fear persecution. As a brown-skinned Muslim woman, she now lived under threat and suspicion. Our differences unconsciously registered in the first session.

Ms A. arrived five minutes late to her first session. When I greeted her in the waiting room, she walked past me into the office and muttered, "Damn these trains." She came into the office speaking in great detail about the tubes in London, which were much superior to NYC subways. She left no space for introductions.

> I am not the kind of person who comes late or gets lost, which is why I am late. I have superior spatial relations; I never get lost. These idiots who are worried about the subway being blown up, they should. The way this system is built, there is no way it could be protected.

I recall being taken aback by what on the surface seemed impersonal, but her level of defensiveness and accusation must have condensed with the heightened awareness of a city defined by code orange, a high-level threat, and the subway as target. Ms A. in a state of accusation that entered the field very fast, I heard a barrage of confrontational questions about myself related to my clinical orientation, training, how long a typical therapy is, and how long I'd been practicing. I fought through a state of withdrawal, probably based in feeling attacked, and realised that she was questioning me with great suspicion. Since Ms A. took over the treatment space very quickly, I had to locate and balance myself in the context of accusation and find a way to connect with her. This went on for several sessions as I struggled to hold my own experience and not be defensive, until Ms A. let her guard down enough to allow me to understand something about her reasons for seeking help. She had become argumentative and impossible to get along with. She said that she had gone overboard, but this domineering, take-charge attitude worked for her professionally as the director of a non-profit agency with a global mission.

Over the course of the first year, the stability of the frame and a manifest trust developed that was based in some of our shared realities that we both reached into. Ms A. and I were close in age and shared a sociopolitical orientation that was based in an implicit understanding that I empathised with her struggles as a mother of school-aged children immersed in a professional life that was meaningful to her. As the treatment deepened, I began to attend to the particular ways that Ms A. spoke to me about her staff and how poorly they carried out her mandates. Her disdain paralleled her experience of the poorly structured subways. Ms A. was condescending, rigid, and within an increasingly tense treatment space, I became increasingly aware that my thinking was met with frustration and increasing intolerance. I was able to talk to her about the ways in which she was turning me into someone of little value.

As the summer break approached, Ms A. came to a session muttering to herself and cursing her support staff. Shaking her head from side to side, she covered her eyes and was clearly unable to manage. I said that I could see how lost she had become in frustration and anger. She continued under her breath, "Support staff, stupid White girls, why is everyone so afraid of me? Do they still think I am going to blow up the subway?" Ms A. lifted her head and glared at me. I held the provocation, which falsely depicted her as the one inflicting terror and said that I could now understand more about the dangers she felt from others. No wonder she was so on edge. She replied, "Americans are stupid." I told her that she wanted me to not be stupid and notice that she was in a vulnerable position as a Muslim woman, post 9/11. She paused, and we both relaxed. Ms A. then told me of whispers she overheard at her daughter's school, white parents saying, "[T]hey are among us." She spoke about transferring her daughter to a more diverse school. As I listened, I recognised that the tensions I had felt in sessions had lessened. Having acknowledged racialisation in the field, I no longer felt like the white, American enemy, and Ms A. was able to whisper her vulnerabilities and talk about how unprotected she felt as a Muslim woman. We thought about her anger and condescension as a personality trait that protected her from all the accusatory looks in her white neighbourhood. Ms A.'s associations led to terror, the subway, and a memory, not one that she ever thought had much significance, of being told that her mother's family was hidden "underground" during a state-mandated police raid. Encompassing the analytic field in a frightening post-9/11 world was an unconscious of hiding underground that was linked in the present to the tubes, the subway, representing secrecy and whispers to take protective measures and hide. Ms A. had thought of women from her native origins as submissive and naïve, relied on only for traditional function; she began to consider how thoughtful her mother and women of her generation had to be to avoid assault.

Ms A. and I came to understand the defensive function of her aggressiveness as a disidentification from a false narrative about women. I learned that like me, her mother had light skin. Light-skinned women from her origins were considered beautiful but seen as passive. Ms A. equated her dark skin with her father, who was highly educated.

Over the next month we were able to process how anger and condescension served as a defence. Ms A.'s achievements did not protect her from the dangers associated with racism. Like her mother, and the many generations of women before her, she learned that acceptance of vulnerability lead to thinking and resourcefulness. Ms A.'s gendered narrative expanded through a field where we both participated. The politicised narrative of terrorism exposed a deepened contact with a racist narrative that permeated the city. The condescension and anger evidenced the impact of a broadened field, a post-9/11 world that entered the analytic space. The trauma of the present allowed us to hear the "whisper" of transmitted trauma, *après-coup*, now, through an expanded psychic reality.

Life in the Death Instinct: COVID-19

Mr M., an Orthodox Jewish man now in his sixties had been improving with analysis before the pandemic started. He originally came to treatment after his doctors found no medical evidence for somatic events that would lead to fainting spells and palpitations. Over the years he has needed analysis to help him represent mental states rather than erase his mind, hold pain in his body, or act out his rage through alcohol abuse. Mr M. suffered early trauma in connection with a life-threatening medical illness when he was four. For complex reasons related to a familial Holocaust history, Mr M. was offered very little containment by his parents, both of whom had limited capacity to understand mental suffering because of their own traumas. In childhood, as an Orthodox Jew, he was subjected to bullying, and this in combination with continued experiences of parental mis-attunement, led to Mr M. developing an oppositional character. When he was not fighting, he would swallow his rage and submit. Over years in analysis, he worked through rage and unmet dependency needs in the transference sand was beginning to work through his unconscious belief that my having a separate mind was not an attack on him. The intersubjective field space was constructed around tolerance for communication, separateness, and beginning ownership of psychic pain.

When COVID-19 entered the immediate surround in NYC, residents retreated into the new world of quarantine. Link-NYC, a cutting-edge digital communication network that posts news stories, cultural events, and inspiration, all over the city, suddenly, converted their signage and symbols to represent the new pandemic order: "Flatten the Curve, Stop the Spread, 6-Feet- Apart, Wear a Face Covering." Mr M. became increasingly sceptical of the virus and the public health order to close offices and move to online work. Mr M. became increasingly cynical, acerbic, and soon enough attacking of the analyst for participating in the public health initiative. He regressed to living in a state of argument, and his capacity for flexible thought and uncertainty collapsed. He became consumed with conspiracy theories related to the government's exaggeration of the virus, providing statistics that this was no different than the flu. He believed that COVID-19 was used as a decoy for political gains. The field space was taken over by his omnipotent ideas, manic denial, and complete intolerance of separateness. In sessions, he projectively forced his terrors of a government takeover into me. If I in any way validated his beliefs, particularly if I indicated any reservations about NYC officials and their handling of the pandemic, he would panic. I was to uphold an authoritative stance that he could rage against. It would become clear that I was to hold his fears of being taken over by his unconscious destructive wishes, represented by COVID and its death force.

While there were obvious connections between the pandemic and Mr M.'s early encounters with death, his obsession with the political divisions around COVID-19 remained hyperreal and inaccessible to thought or dream.

When the COVID-19 vaccines became accessible, Mr M. became more ensconced in his beliefs, producing evidence that the pharmaceutical companies were concealing serious risks from the public. Mr M. confronted me about whether I received the vaccine, and when I told him in a voice that must have conveyed my enormous gratitude, I sensed, even over the phone, that he had calmed down for the first time in months. A long silence followed. Mr M. said that he had drifted into a thought maybe a memory, a fantasy, he was not sure. He talked about his shared excitement with his father when in 1969 the NY Mets won the world series. This was an experience that I shared with my father as a child and, now in an emotional moment, understood that Mr M. was talking about the miracle of a losing team, battling to win and succeeding. Mr M. recalled his father lifting him in the air, and he felt like a winner. He had never seen his father joyous, but now, après-coup, understood that the Mets winning represented hope and life for both of them. For that moment, the father's deadness, based in all the dehumanisation and traumatic loss that he had experienced in the camps, had evaporated enough for my patient to feel love. He believed that this freed him from the terror of his own childhood illness and facilitated his fighting spirit. My communication of gratitude for the vaccine brought life into a repetitive and dead analytic field. I believe that my taking action to protect myself relieved Mr M. from his unconscious phantasies of destructiveness and enlivened him. A series of dreams about his father followed that permitted mourning and remembrance. While Mr M. remains deeply sceptical of COVID-19 and the vaccine, his panic and emphatic denial has lessened and seems to have opened the analysis again to an acceptance of difference and a greater capacity for empathy.

Conclusion

Analytic field theory encompasses a broad spectrum of psychoanalytic thought that offers an expanded dimension to hold and listen for the dimensioned complexities of transmitted trauma in a present context. In addition to the internal situation, psychic structure and psychic reality are shaped by intergenerational history and influenced by the sociocultural elements of the immediate surround. In the clinical cases discussed, the field is influenced by extreme events in the immediate surround of New York City, 9/11 and COVID-19, which produced a heightened experience of threat, impacting the shape and development of the analytic dyad within an intersubjective space. Each patient brought psychic experiences to the treatment that evidenced an unconscious life interfaced with a world of "othering." A presentation of defensive posturing concealed vulnerabilities that found a place in the transference-countertransference field. On the analyst's side of the dyad, opportunities to build a creative intersubjective space emerged from understanding how the environmental context, while not always as extreme as 9/11 and COVID-19, ignited unconscious alienation from an internal parent whose trauma was remembered and found in an intersubjective emotional moment with the analyst.

The development of the field is reliant on the analyst's capacity to develop a narrative that is attentive to the patient's inner and outer worlds, while searching for the echoes of intergenerational history. Psychoanalysis is expanding the lens of field, integrating the impact of a traumatic history on generational violence. As psychoanalysis continues to confront its own intergenerational trauma, disavowed racism and racialisation will be thought about in clinical practice and included as a dimension in theory. Social structures that degrade differences need to be listened to more closely in the clinical situation and understood temporally. Freud (1923) posited that the unconscious is timeless, and while the traces of the repressed are permanent, the capacity to bear trauma and mentalise pain offers potential for psychic growth.

References

Akhtar, S. (1999). The immigrant, the exile, and the experience of nostalgia. *Journal of Applied Psychoanalytic Studies, 1,* 123–130.

Apprey, M. (2017). Representing, theorizing and reconfiguring the concept of trans-generational hauntings in order to facilitate healing. In S. Grand & J. Salberg (Eds.), *Trans-generational trauma and the other: Dialogues across history and difference.* New York, NY: Routledge and Taylor & Francis Group.

Baranger, M., & Baranger, W. (2008). The analytic situation as a dynamic field. *The International Journal of Psychoanalysis, 89*(4), 795–826.

Bion, W. R. (1962). *Learning from experience.* London: Karnac Books.

Faimberg, H. (1996). Listening to listening. *International Journal of Psychoanalysis. 77*(Pt. 4), 667–677.

Faimberg, H., (2005). *The telescoping of generations: Listening to the narcissistic links between generations.* London: Routledge.

Ferro, A., & Civitarese, G. (2019). *Analytic field and its transformations.* London: Routledge.

Freud, S. (1923). *The ego and the Id.* The Standard Edition of the Complete Psychological Works of Sigmund Freud, Volume XIX. London: Hogarth Press.

Grand, S., & Salberg, J. (2017). *Trans-generational trauma and the other: Dialogues across history and difference.* New York, NY: Routledge and Taylor & Francis Group.

Leary, K. (1997). Race in psychoanalytic space. *Gender and Psychoanalysis, 2,* 157–172.

Mitchell, S. A., Aron, L., Harris, A., & Suchet, M. (Eds.). (1999). *Relational psychoanalysis.* Hillsdale, NJ: Analytic Press.

Holmes, D. E. (1992). Race in the transference in psychoanalysis and psychotherapy. *International Journal of Psychoanalysis, 73*–11.

Holmes, D. E. (2016). Culturally imposed trauma: The sleeping dog has awakened. Will psychoanalysis take heed? *Psychoanalytic Dialogues, 26,* 641–654.

Katz, M., & Civitarese, G. (2017). *Advances in contemporary psychoanalytic field theory: Concept and future development.* London: Routledge.

Moss, D. (2021, April). On having whiteness. *Journal of the American Psychoanalytic Association, 69*(2), 355–371.

Powell, D. R. (2018). Race, African Americans, and psychoanalysis: Collective silence in the therapeutic encounter. *Journal of the American Psychoanalytic Association, 66,* 6.

Renik, O. (1999). *Relational psychoanalysis, volume 2: Innovation and expansion.* Retrieved March 15, 2022, from www.readallbooks.org/book/relational-psychoanalysis-volume-2-innovation-and-expansion/.

Silverman, M. A. (2017). On the birth and development of psychoanalytic field theory, Part 2. *Psychoanalytic Quarterly, 86,* 919–932.

Stoute, J. (2017, Winter/Spring). Race and racism in psychoanalytic thought: The ghosts in our nursery. *American Psychoanalyst, Quarterly Magazine of the American Psychoanalytic Association, 51*(1).

Suchet, M. (2007). Unraveling whiteness. *Psychoanalytic Dialogues, 17*(6), 867–886.

Winnicott, D. W. (1953). Transitional objects and transitional phenomena; A study of the first not-me possession. *The International Journal of Psychoanalysis, 34,* 89–97.

Winnicott, D. W. (1956). On transference. *International Journal of Psychoanalysis, 37,* 386–388.

Woods, A. (2020). The work before us: Whiteness at the psychoanalytic institute. *Psychoanalysis, Culture & Society, 25*(2), 230–249.

8 Psychoanalysis and the drama of refugees in Italy

Fabio Castriota

The psychoanalysis and the drama of the refugees

Forty-four years ago, an international congress titled "Psychic Traumatisation through Social Catastrophe" was held in Copenhagen, and the issues discussed then are still dramatically relevant today. In these years, already 100,000 refugees have sought asylum in Europe, most landing on the Italian coastline from 2010. Related to these migratory flows which bring human beings in conditions of threatened survival to the old continent are events such as war, persecution, or extreme conditions of existence. This challenges us, not merely as citizens but as psychoanalysts as well. The Mediterranean Sea, a cradle of civilisation, the Romans' *mare nostrum*, has turned into a place of despair and everyday tragedy, a vast cemetery of broken lives. Already 1,000 people have perished in 2021 and 18,000 in the last ten years!

Trying to address this humanitarian crisis by offering its own contribution, the SPI Executive launched the PER Project Working Group (PER stands for European Psychoanalysts for Refugees in Italian) in March 2016. I am glad to have been able to serve as group coordinator in my capacity as SPI vice president.

We set to work with these two guidelines:

1) The development of a psychoanalytic reflection on migratory events. Deep-seated emotional responses have been aroused within the resident populations of Europe to the confrontation with tragedy of the new arrivals as asylum seekers and their psychosocial culture. Our perspective is to increase awareness of these issues.
2) Our direct participation is to become part of specific projects, providing training for volunteer and practitioner groups, through international bidding applications together with other European societies.

Psychoanalysis and migrants: a possible encounter?

My first topic will consider the possibility of extending the methodology of psychoanalysis to the analysis of the issues affecting migrant populations

DOI: 10.4324/9781003203223-10

from a non-European cultural background. Our own position stems from the idea that the method of psychoanalysis is quite suitable for an in-depth understanding of the issues presented by people uprooted from their cultural context. These people are without an anchor in this fundamental psychic matrix that is the symbolisation apparatus. It is because of this outlook that the psychoanalytical method appears particularly relevant for the comprehension of the dimensions of "passing through," transition, and transformation, for the necessity of their comprehension.

The migratory phenomenon

As is well known, migratory transit flows see the activation of a deep-seated sense of precariousness as well as the transformation of these meta-psychic and meta-social frames of reference described by Kaës (2007). The function of these frames of reference is to stabilise repressing agencies, narcissistic constructs, and the genealogies which build up bonds and meaning. This primary relationship is deeply affected by such destabilising effects, and it is there that the farthest-reaching and most concealed fractures of the migratory phenomenon bury themselves. Rethinking the maternal function in the light of migratory transit flows, as well as the crucial issues of origins, transgenerational transference, and the paternal function, all represent areas of fundamental importance. Likewise, the notions of "borders" and of "working on borders" – psychic, relational, and cultural borders – become of primary importance in this perspective.

The most frequent issues arising in these extreme situations, however, remain: i) what Lifton (1970) has called "the stigma of death" – the with an anxiety-laden search for meaning, under the dominion of a death-anxiety which threatens to destroy the self; iii) a psychic numbing which leads to the loss of the capacity to feel, as if the refugee underwent a symbolic death in order to avoid the final psychic and physical destruction; iv) various and contrasting conflicts between desires for intimacy, reliance, and nourishment, mingled with resentment for the help received while fearing renewed loss. Anger may become, in some cases, a desperate striving to feel alive and escape innermost death. The refugee may thus end up feeling remote and isolated, while in fear of the company of otherness. Feeling different, refugees become isolated or relate only to those who share a similar trauma. This is the reason why the earliest sign of recovery is to be found in a renewed search for others who differ from the self.

The encounter between the therapist and the migrant

First and foremost, the therapist is called upon to "think through" the fracture I was referring to earlier. In a certain sense as well, this is a call to dream without withdrawing from that "lost feeling" which comes alive in a transcultural relationship while we are coming to grips with its symbolic configurations. As we know, one finds oneself involved in these relationships with an investment overload of the perceptive channels which literally overflow with signs and signals from sensory differences – those differences being insufficiently linked to shared symbolic representations.

For this very reason, these relationships are paradoxically much more marked by excess rather than want, and this explains why a phobic avoidance reaction is often triggered, from which stems the sensation of the impossibility of establishing a therapeutic setting.

Another major point is the analysis of the fractures that are generated within the central functions of the primary relationships. What does indeed happen when facing these conditions of cultural discontinuity? Piera Aulagnier (2001) underscores that, as long as one remains within the bounds of one's own culture, the mother can efficaciously carry out her role of mouthpiece for her child. When, however, the mother must function in a cultural system to which she may not herself belong at all, it is that central function itself which becomes disarticulated. This places the very use of the instrument of language as the fundamental medium of symbolisation of the primary affect experience at risk.

Besides, we should never forget that it is above all among the modalities of transgenerational psychic and cultural transference that the most lacerating effects of the migratory experience come to lurk. For it is in these situations that we end up finding that the possibility of assigning a child the role of offspring – the possibility of affiliation to one's own lineage, one's chain of ascendants and symbolic memberships – to be deeply compromised. It is on a genealogical plane, therefore, that the fracture which will have multiple consequences, specifically on the narcissistic underpinnings of the feeling of identity. Thus, in these circumstances, a traumatic event not only divides the continuity of the sense of self but also the fabric of group membership, the basic bond between self and other. It is the basal connective tissue that is ruptured, and the essential basis of survival which is undermined. To elaborate this trauma, promoting only symbolisation work is not sufficient, as the violation of the inter-human bond has involved every bond, and thus also the analyst who, as a subject, has in turn undergone, and been forced to elaborate, the same violation as any member of the human community. In these contexts, the therapeutic function is primarily that of a presence, of sharing, of witnessing, carried out through listening and confirming that the communication has been received.

The emotional and phantasmal impact of these situations, therefore, cannot be but overwhelming and perturbing, as encounters and images of people whose survival is being threatened bring back into play some experiences of our lives to a primal level, this fundamental unconscious substrate awaiting symbolisation which is known to us from birth. An immediate reaction would be to avert our gaze from these children that we, too, were once, and from these conditions of desperate helplessness, of dependence on others.

The rootless uproot, Hannah Arendt (1958) wrote, and contact with those who bear the signs of traumatic uprooting upon their person does not leave onlookers untouched, it relentlessly keeps on uprooting whatever comes close. Nietzsche (1886) reminds us that, if we gaze into the abyss, the abyss will stare back into our eyes. The widespread and instinctive perception that migrants bring disorder and confusion evinces the traumatic nature of the contact, which has an unknown component because the outline, the image, and the very reference grid for thinking contacts has been mislaid. An emergency is therefore always associated with the unthought-of, that for which a domain of thought is still lacking and remains to be found: something for which some thinking space will have to be found. In the transition from anxiety to a relationship with the extraneous, we massively and instinctively recruit psychosomatic areas of an archaic nature. This has to do with the necessity to assume the other within our own psyche/soma, to have an experience of the other which involves the sensory, the emotions, and even the drives (in the broad sense of the term). This is precisely because the symbolic means of elaboration of an unconscious emergency – understood as arousal – as well as phantasmal expectation, cannot be shared. Those(?) will make themselves heard by literally invading the field of both intra- and inter-psychic experiences, hence the widespread perception of a conquest of the field of the thinkable. This is what relentlessly pushes towards various modalities of discharge through action.

The migrant and the practitioner

We cannot speak about the subjective experience of a refugee without thinking about this refugee being in a dyad with an aid worker: the intensity and the quality of the emotional experiences at play is only there in the flow of complex interactions that can be communicated in the dialogical and behavioural dynamics of this dyad. It is similar to the mother-infant experience and is as intense and without the mediation of speech. Primary symbolisation work requires the activation of this capacity for openness towards unconscious communication, which is part of the psychoanalyst's preparedness. This capacity is particularly valuable in the work with aid workers who are often overwhelmed by the violent nature of the traumatic misadventures of the refugees. From this perspective, we cannot speak of the subjective experience of a refugee without thinking of this refugee as in a dyad with an aid worker, just as we cannot think of the subjective/professional experience of an aid worker without reference to a refugee aid operation.

The psychoanalytical method has significant instruments to offer. The institution of sufficiently stable settings to establish a minimum of continuity and address migrant and aid worker connected issues represents a valuable resource. It partly interrupts precariousness in the background and establishes a psychic locus where experiences that migrants and analysts have encountered and lived through can be collected and where their intensity can become meaningful.

A possible response, therefore, could be the creation of working and training groups for the purpose of investigating and responding through new forms of symbolisation with the involvement of images, words, and stories which speak for this unprecedented new world.

In this context, the supervisor's function as a mental third is essential, as it can generate a specific whirlwind of analytical listening within the group of aid workers who listen to each other through the listening of the analyst. The construction of the "encounter space" is essential and preliminary to any possible functioning of thought: this is the necessary definition of a setting which is even more necessary since it has been endlessly and constantly criticised. It is the specific quality of the analytical listening that can activate a form of psychic metabolisation among witnesses who may later be able to pick up their traces, slowly and painstakingly, and even among survivors. Living in close contact with survivors is one of the most difficult experiences to elaborate and to manage without being oneself devastated by it. It is fundamental to be capable of living silently next to people while being capable of waiting that an authentic discourse on the horror they have lived might emerge from their silence. There is the necessity of a slow-paced and deep-reaching reconstruction of the fabric of their everyday life. Living in the proximity of migrants requires a special tolerance of a regimen of minimal emotional investments – at worst, of non-investment, that lasts the whole time it can take for a mind in survival mode to tolerate this turning back to life. This is why such a function can only be taken up by aid workers who build together with their guests a shared space for everyday living. Moreover, they must accept not to crowd this space to excess (with objects but also with "affects," etc.) or scarcity. Thus, it is essential that the workers should be helped to tolerate the necessity for the survivors to remain stuck in the "inhumanity" of their ordeal. Alternatively, they can be helped to visualise what havoc "relocating" into an ordered way of life can wreak in people who have had to adapt to chaos and a violent existence. They must be shown that their very survival depended on their capacity to adapt. Violent integration anxiety attacks can develop on this path back towards humanity, but also instinctual emergencies can occur for which aid administrations show scant tolerance.

In conclusion, what working with migrants requires from us is to be ever more thoroughly psychoanalysts. This is through a renewed, profound engagement of our listening to what is most extraneous to us. Great staying power in our negative capability, which is sorely tested, is also required, together with a constant aptitude for self-analysis. We need this to be able to bring into play our own traumatised, unvoiced, and submerged areas, areas of trauma, areas which we may not have analysed in ourselves and which, for that reason, remain particularly disturbing and difficult to contact.

Possible forms of intervention

Among various initiatives throughout Europe, the instrument of the clinical group seminars has a specific indication and is currently the most commonly used training instrument in the borderland where aid workers are constantly exposed to burnout. It is a space where the pervasive anxiety experienced in their everyday work can be unburdened, where stability is essential, where there is a pre-scheduled time dedicated to the transformation processes of the mental states of the participants. Its analytical quality consists in the elements which characterise its methodology: a well-defined setting and an approach based on free associations from the participants and the evenly floating attention of a leader who, following an intense interplay of conscious/unconscious interventions between group members must piece together the various aspects of the case that the participants have grasped in the discussion. In its functioning through free associations and floating attention, the group realises the resumption of the functioning of the thinking apparatus as an oscillation between emotion, action, and the analytic specificity of knowledge. The essential requirement is to widen the psychic functioning in which knowledge has also become the object. It is a self-transformative process, not only an observational one.

A narrative function is thus activated, finding ways to give shape and meaning to what happens by rescuing it from a one-way fate as the evacuating action of a discharge. The curative and thinking function are enacted by the group itself, of which the aid worker who presented the crisis situation that arose from his work with refugees as well as the psychoanalyst leader are members. Viewed from this perspective, the clinical seminar is an instance of transformative learning: it enables an understanding of aspects of the work relation situation that could not have been grasped by the individual dimension of one mind on its own. It triggers a transformation of the emotional state of the participants who, in turn, are called upon to become characters of the inner world that is presented and function as split off aspects, which are denied and are not represented, while they are put into action by unconscious group dynamics. Through emotional exposure, group members signify their own availability to house the extraneous, the other than themselves, to let unknown aspects of themselves emerge, without individual analytic interpretations in view.

In conclusion, I would like to say that the functioning aspects of this experience can be summed up by the following dimensions: constructing a setting, listening, suffering, associating, and configuring. The ultimate goal remains to help others rebuild the meaning of their personal experience, give back a sense to their trauma and hope in their life.

References

Arendt, H. (1958). *The human condition*. Chicago: University of Chicago Press.

Aulagnier, P. (2001). *The violence of interpretation*. The New Library of Psychoanalysis. London: Brunner-Routledge.

Kaës, R. (2007). *Un singulier pluriel*. Malakoff, France: Dunond.

Lifton, R. J. (1970). *History and human survival*. New York: Random House.

Nietzsche, F. (1886), *Jenseits von Gut und Böse*, Alfred Körner Verlag. Leipzig.

9 Mourning and issues of identity in the treatment of refugees in Lesvos

Anna L Christopoulos, Chrysi Giannoulaki, and Nicholas Tzavaras

Introduction: The Refugee Crisis in Greece

The refugee crisis in Europe has constituted the biggest wave of migration since World War II (Doctors of the World, 2021a). The majority of arrivals have come from countries involved in wars, thus fleeing violence, persecution, torture, even death. Greece has been the main gateway to Europe, and more than 1.5 million asylum seekers have passed through Greece since 2014 (Operational Data Portal, 2021). According to the UNHCR report of May 2021, 89,000 people received international protection in Greece between January 2016 and April 2021. A number of islands in Greece are the initial point of entry including Chios, Kos, Samos, and Leros, although the main entry point is the island of Lesvos-Mytilini (Doctors of the World, 2021b). In the most recent survey of a total of 800 migrants and refugees, 91% of new arrivals said the main reason they travelled to Greece was "to escape violence" (Efstathiou, 2021).

From the beginning, the refugee crisis has drawn the attention of the entire world (Lijtmaer, 2017). In Greece, the international response was massive as world leaders and celebrities visited the camps, while ordinary citizens from across the globe came to volunteer their services in their particular areas of expertise such as medicine and law. Some simply volunteered wherever they were needed. Several documentaries were made including *4.1 Miles* (Daphne Matziaraki, 2016), which won a 2016 Peabody Award and was nominated for a 2017 Academy Award about a Hellenic Coast Guard captain on Lesvos charged with the task of saving thousands of people crossing the Aegean Sea, and *No Human is Illegal* (Ledes, 2019) based on interviews of asylum seekers in the camp of Moria on the island of Lesvos.

The initial response of Greek citizens to the arrival of asylum seekers was overwhelmingly positive, with people from all walks of life donating money, food, and volunteering wherever they could to help (Kalantzakos, 2017). According to a 2016 poll, two out of three Greeks responded that they feel compassion and sadness for asylum seekers who had arrived (Public Issue, 2016). Many people went out of their way to offer what

DOI: 10.4324/9781003203223-11

they could to the new arrivals. Six out of ten Greeks polled reported that they had contributed in donating food (39%), clothing (31%), medical supplies and sanitation supplies (11%), monies (10%), children's toys (7%), and supplies such as tents and blankets. This was particularly striking given that the majority of people were facing severe financial hardships, as Greece was in a severe austerity program. Moreover, a study of semistructured interviews revealed that many citizens volunteered to help in various capacities, particularly after the closing of the northern border (Kalantzakos, 2017). Unfortunately, the situation for asylum seekers in Greece deteriorated over time. The lack of coordination and poor management of funds resulted in severe overcrowding in many camps leading to problematic, even dangerous living conditions characterized by poor sanitation and crime (Amnesty International, 2020; Das, 2018). The government response has also been internationally criticized for its border policies (World Report, 2021). Interestingly, however, according to the most recent poll, when asked, 65% of asylum seekers chose the words "gratitude" and 56% the word "love" to describe their feelings towards the Greek population who received them (Efstathiou, 2021).

The Hellenic Psychoanalytic Society has attempted to contribute to the relief effort in a number of ways from the beginning of the crisis. Several members, as well as analysts in training have key administrative positions in NGOs for asylum seekers, while others work in clinical capacities including psychiatric intervention, psychodynamically oriented psychotherapy therapy, supervision, and training. In addition, several members, including the current authors collaborated in a group based on the work of the NGO *Doctors of the World*, with the participation of the Psychology department of the University of Athens, and the Hellenic Psychiatric Association. The group conducted a series of qualitative research studies with asylum seekers with the aim of understanding all aspects of their experience. In addition, some members of the group worked in a supervisory and therapeutic capacity with asylum seekers.

Psychoanalysis and the Current Refugee Crisis

The response of the psychoanalytic community throughout the world to refugees during the last years has been notable. Particularly in Europe and in the United States, analysts have engaged in clinical work with refugees. In addition, a significant number of clinical and theoretical studies have focused on exploring the complex, multidimensional experiences of asylum seekers as well as considering approaches to intervention (eg, Leuzinger-Bohleber & Hettich, 2018; Luci & Kahn, 2021; Orfanos, 2019; Togashi & Brothers, 2021; Zarnegar & Mohammadpour-Yazdi, 2021). This is particularly significant given that, until recently, psychoanalytic study of asylum seekers had been neglected (Sperry & Mull, 2021; Volkan, 2017). The current interest in this area is clearly in recognition of the fact that forced migration can lead to significant mental suffering (Abou-Saleh & Chistodoulou, 2016; Ben Farhat et al., 2018; Luci & Kahn, 2021; Morina et al., 2018; Poole et al., 2018). Moreover, it has also been noted that post-migration conditions can have an equally significant positive effects on post-migration adaptation (Leuzinger-Bohleber & Hettich, 2018). In a recent meta-analysis of studies to date, various factors in the post-migration environment were shown to be of critical importance regarding the adjustment of asylum seekers, thus underlining the significance of intervention after the arrival of the asylum seeker to the first place of entry (Jannesari et al., 2020).

Psychoanalytic study of the refugee crisis to date has focused on a number of significant areas. The traumatic dimensions of the experience of asylum seekers have been underscored. Forced uprooting from the homeland, horrific experiences such as exposure to extreme violence, witnessing of death, unprecedented terror, separation from family and other loved ones, and conditions of extreme physical and mental deprivation are typical. According to Cohen, these are "psychotic experiences anchored in reality events" (Cohen & Wills, 1985, p. 310).

As noted by Varvin (2017) the psychoanalytic approach to trauma is particularly critical, in juxtaposition to the application of the concept of trauma in the general mental health literature regarding asylum seekers. Within psychoanalysis, the trauma, by definition, specifically involves the flooding of the psyche with unbearable stimulation and experience leading to severe difficulties in mental representation of capacities and symbolization (Lijtmaer, 2017; Luci & Kahn, 2021; Varvin, 2016, 2017, 2019). As a result, the traumatic experiences of asylum seekers are dissociated, engraved on the body, resulting in a series of somatic complaints, or as overwhelming thoughts and feelings and behaviours (Beritzhoff, 2021; Luci & Kahn, 2021; Varvin, 2017). Mental traces or fragments of traumatic experiences appear in the form of disturbing dreams, somatic sensations, or even hallucinations (Nutting, 2019; Varvin, 2017). While these phenomena are typically viewed as pathological from the general mental health community and treated with medication, the psychoanalytic approach sees these as manifestations of the human response to overwhelming inhuman stress requiring psychological interventions, with some even calling the ethics of medicalizing these symptoms into question (Achotegui, 2019; Nutting, 2019).

The mourning process has also been underscored as particularly significant for refugees (Achotegui, 2019; Akhtar, 1999; Beritzhoff, 2021; Volkan, 2017). In a recent article Achotegui (2019) distinguishes between simple mourning, which occurs under favourable conditions; complicated mourning, in cases where there are serious difficulties in working through migratory grief; and extreme mourning, where this grief cannot be resolved. He proposes the concept of the "Ulysses syndrome" to describe the latter, which is characteristic of the mourning process of immigrants. Symptoms include sadness, tension, irritability, insomnia, recurrent and intrusive thoughts, disorientation, depersonalization, and derealization, as well as the aforementioned somatic symptoms such as migraines, osteoarticular complaints, and fatigue. In his view, understanding of the Ulysses syndrome helps the clinician avoid an incorrect diagnosis of depressive, psychotic, or antisocial disorders in immigrants. Cultural dimensions of the person's experience and symptomatology have been noted to be of critical significance. The individual's interpretation of these symptoms based on his own cultural experiences is characteristic, as, for example, the view that the current troubles are a result of bad luck or witchcraft (Luci & Kahn, 2021, p. 202; Stitou, 2021).

Psychoanalytically based interventions are multidimensional given the complexity of the refugee situation. The creation of a containing environment, with initial individual consultations and later individual and group psychotherapies has been found to be very useful. Basic goals are the creation of a sense of trust in another, the possibility of beginning to give voice to external and internal experience leading to amelioration of internal fragmentation and re-establishment of the mentalizing function as well as more secure models of relationships (Leuzinger-Bohleber, 2018; Leuzinger-Bohleber et al., 2016; Varvin, 2019). In time, when longer-term intervention is possible, therapy may enable recognition and understanding of painful object relational mechanisms and dynamics such as projections, unconscious conflicts, and fantasies, as well as libidinal and aggressive impulses. Modification of classical psychoanalytic and psychotherapeutic technique is indicated in view of the particularly traumatic nature of the refugee experience (Leuzinger-Bohleber et al., 2016; Oliner, 2014; Bohleber & Leuzinger-Bohleber, 2016). Transference and countertransference developments often take specific forms such as non-verbal, bodily manifestations, and enactments (Luci & Kahn, 2021; Varvin, 2019).

However, in many contexts, external reality permits only very short-term interventions at best, which can nonetheless be of notable value (Jović, 2018; Nutting, 2019). Camps are often overwhelmed beyond capacity and understaffed, leading clinicians to resort to the use of medication solely to address the problems presented by asylum seekers. The camp of Moria on the island of Lesvos in Greece is a case in point. Moria has been the subject of international focus and severe criticism, after a *New York Times* article in 2018 published an interview with Dr Alessandro Barberio, the chief psychiatrist of the NGO *Doctors without Borders* (Kingsley, 2016). In this interview, besides condemning the abysmal and dangerous living conditions of the camp, Dr Barberio reported that his staff was able to treat the majority of those asking for help only with antipsychotic medication. This tendency has been confirmed by psychoanalytically oriented clinicians volunteering at the camp

(Beritzhoff, 2021; Nutting, 2019). However, for these analysts, the importance of offering time to those asking for help, however limited that time might be, was seen as of paramount importance given that listening, characterized by empathy, bearing witness to and accepting the experiences of the traumatized is a first step in healing trauma (Beritzhoff, 2021; Lijtmaer, 2017; Luci & Kahn, 2021). This was even more the case since many asylum seekers had not been able to speak to anyone about their experiences and feelings.

Many of these dimensions of the psychoanalytic approach regarding understanding of and intervention with refugees may be seen in the following vignette of a brief intervention, comprising three sessions, with Mr A., an asylum seeker, and the second author, a psychiatrist and psychoanalyst of the Hellenic Psychoanalytic Society who was working in the Camp of Moria in Lesvos.

Mr A.

Mr A., a 25-year-old African man from the Congo was referred to me for psychiatric evaluation two weeks after arriving at the camp, as he had reported that he heard voices talking to him that frightened him. Thus, there was concern that he might be in a psychotic episode. I considered that a differential diagnosis was indicated given that these symptoms are not necessarily pathognomonic of psychosis with this severely traumatized group of people. He was also reported to be irritable and aggressive with those around him, behaviours that were, in my experience, characteristic of many asylum seekers in this camp.

My initial impression of Mr A. when he came in, was of an attractive, likable young man. He made good and steady eye contact, which immediately gave me a sense of relief, as it was a contraindication of psychosis. His good posture and well-coordinated body movements were also in line with less severe pathology. Moreover, he spoke with ease through the interpreter who was present throughout the first interview.

When asked about how he was feeling, Mr A. readily replied that he had a great deal of difficulty sleeping and that his body hurt in many places. I knew that these symptoms were very common with asylum seekers in the camp, as bodily pain appears to be the way that many can experience internal pain resulting from their traumatic experiences. Mr A. had fled from his village after soldiers suddenly burst into his house and killed everyone in his family in front of him. He was one of the few to escape, as most were killed. In this first interview, Mr A. also reported that he heard ghosts – that is, dead people – talking to him not only when he was asleep but throughout the day, which was extremely frightening for him. I was thus faced with the question of whether these voices were verbal hallucinations or whether they were flashback experiences of the traumatic events he had lived through. There was also a question of whether the bodily pain in multiple sites was within the framework of posttraumatic stress disorder or hypochondriacal symptoms signifying the beginning of a psychosis.

After discussion of his pain symptoms, Mr A. spontaneously returned to talking about the ghosts. He stated they were "wild" and thus scared him a great deal. I considered it a positive sign that Mr A. wanted to talk about the ghosts and brought up this topic himself again, as this was another contraindication of psychosis. In my experience, psychotic individuals usually tend to hide or avoid talking about their hallucinatory symptoms. However, his need to talk about these experiences also indicated to me that they were important and that the internal purpose or meaning of these ghosts for Mr A. needed to be understood. Spontaneously what came to my mind associatively was what had been a very significant supervision in the past in my work with a patient who saw ghosts. My supervisor at that time had underscored the importance of asking the patient what the ghosts did and said. In a similar vein, the film *The Sixth Sense* also came to my mind, which had included the idea that ghosts that do not stay in the grave are in contact with the living because they need to say something to those left behind.

Thus, I then asked him if he recognized the identity of the ghosts and whether he knew what they were saying to him. Mr A. opened his eyes widely and answered:

> Of course I know them. I have seen many of them die in front of me, relatives and friends and other people I know that were killed after I left my village. However, I don't know what they're saying to me. And I don't want to hear.

My mind also went to the potential cultural aspects of these ghosts – that is, whether they had significance in his particular home environment. However, I was unable to pursue our discussion further because my time to see him had run out for the moment. I noticed that I felt a connection to Mr A., despite the brevity of our meeting, which contributed to my impression that his symptoms were more consistent with a traumatic reaction rather than psychosis. Thus, I told him that I would see him the next week to continue our conversation.

Mr A. was waiting for me when I went to my office the following week. He said he had come earlier than our appointment time, which I understood as an indication that he had found our previous meeting helpful and wanted to see me. Within a few moments I also realized that besides his African dialect he was able to speak in English as can many African asylum seekers. Now able to speak to him directly and without the translator, I asked him how his week had been, and he said that it had been OK but that the ghosts were still around.

I asked him to tell me more details about who those are who are speaking to him as ghosts. I also felt we could now explore the possible cultural dimensions regarding ghosts in his country of origin.

ANALYST: You say that people you knew, who have died talk to you. They have become ghosts. I wonder whether in your village people believe in ghosts, and if so, how they are perceived and dealt with?

MR A.: Of course, we believe in ghosts. Ghosts exist, they talk to us, they eat with us, they're always around us. There are special people who are in a position to talk with them and communicate with them. However, I am very scared because I don't know how to do that. I just want to get rid of them.

His account now brought several thoughts to my mind, all of which revolved around the mourning process. To begin with, I considered that the ghosts represented an attempt to maintain a tie to his home and to his past cultural context. In addition, the ghosts represented those whom Mr A. had lost in a brutal, traumatic manner, people whom he missed but had not yet mourned. I tried to put these thoughts into words.

ANALYST: I understand that you miss those who have died very much. I also think that you miss your country and the way that people there help you to cope with those who have died. I understand that this pain is very great. However, I think that it is important to not get rid of the ghosts, but to see why they are here, what their purpose is. So I suggest that you do the following every time that the ghosts appear – instead of avoiding them, talk with them as much as you can so we can hear and understand together what they are saying to you.

His facial expression changed, he looked very scared, then angry, and almost screamed, "I can't do that," and he looked around in a very frightened manner.

I asked him in what I hoped was a reassuring voice, "Are they here now and are they trying to talk to you?"

MR A.: Yes, they want to tell me all the things that happened to them.

I had a sense of relief once more in my work with this man, as I felt that I was beginning to understand more about the unconscious, inter-psychic dimensions of his experience. I was in the more familiar territory of the mourning process, and the difficulties that are often involved. I considered that he missed his relatives and friends as well as his home and all its cultural dimensions, and the ghosts were a way of retaining contact with him. However, I also thought about his sense of guilt at having survived the lethal attack on his village while these others had not. His need to have these important people from the past tell him what they have gone through was an attempt to expiate his guilt, a reparative effort. I tried to put these thoughts into an interpretation.

ANALYST: You have experienced many painful things, and you feel that you are alone with these experiences. You miss the people that were most important in your life; you wish they were here with you.

MR A. looked relieved and nodded his head as tears came to his eyes.

I continued: So you have the people that you miss come in the form of ghosts to keep you company to talk to you. You want to know what happened to them, to hear how they fared. But maybe because you also feel badly that you left them behind and you were able to come here you are afraid they may be angry with you, so they also scare you.

MR A. again nodded his head and cried more intensely.

MR A.: I wonder whether anyone survived, whether they are somewhere else. And those who didn't, I wonder where they are in the world.

Although I felt pleased with the course of our discussion, I had the sense that there was something that I was missing. I could not identify what this was, but as I allowed my thoughts to wander, I thought about how my sense of him had evolved during our meetings. I had been initially at least somewhat alarmed by the symptoms initially, yet now, as a result of my sense of connection with him, and his clear desire to talk to me, my experience of this man was that he has an underlying strength and desire to survive psychically and to go on with his life. I considered that these transference and countertransference indications might also be related to the appearance of the ghosts. That is, that just as he had the need for me to listen to him, and to hear about his experiences, he similarly wanted those he had to hear what he had been through. Thus, he not only wanted to hear about their experiences, but he had a very strong need for them to hear about his – to know how perilous and agonizing his journey was and how much he had suffered and is suffering. At first glance, I thought that this had to do with his attempt to cope with his profound guilt, for surviving and for abandoning his homeland. I tried to convey this to him as follows.

ANALYST: You want to know about your loved ones and friends, how they are, wherever they are. But I think you also want them to know how you are, where you are, and everything you have been through. So I suggest besides listening to them, you might think of what you want to tell **them**! Talk to them, tell them the things you want them to know. Either when they appear as ghosts, or even just in your thoughts. Tell them about you.

MR A. looks into my eyes intently and questioningly. Nonetheless, I had the strong sense that he wanted to believe me.

ANALYST: I will be here again in one week, and you will come and tell me what you talked about with the ghosts every day. Every time you try to talk to them, try and remember what you said so that you can tell me when we meet again

MR A.: (wonderingly) "Really?"

When I returned the following week, Mr A. seemed much calmer, though very subdued. An air of sadness permeated his expressions and bodily stance. He said that he had talked to the ghosts when they appeared but that they had started to recede and fade away. He had continued the conversation with them "in thought," which made him feel very sad, but I had the sense that the sadness was tolerable for him, an indication that a mourning process had begun.

An additional complexity was that we too now had to separate, as my contact with him was as a consultant, and he would now be working with a therapist. I felt I had little time to address the issue of our separation, which was a repetition of loss, however minor in its form, relative to the losses that he had experienced. It was thus, nonetheless, important to name his disappointment and possible anger at me, to help him in the internalization of a benevolent figure he could talk to as well as to lead the way to the first inklings of the internalization of analytic dialogue with himself.

ANALYST: I think it is very important that you had had these conversations with these loved ones. Many types of conversations, like ours too, can help you. I am sorry that you and I will not be able to talk more. It seems ironic that just had we had started to talk and to know each other, we will have to part. This could make a person sad and angry even a little, especially someone who had been through so much like you have. Here it is, another separation from a person, even though it is someone you have just gotten to know.

MR A. nodded quietly, but said nothing.

I continued. "Someone like me will be able to meet with you for a longer period of time, to talk about all these thoughts and feelings, which may help you feel less afraid of the ghosts, and better in the way that you feel in your life here. It can be sad when people who have had a conversation then have to part, but they can think of each other, and keep the other alive in their mind and heart."

Conclusion

This intervention, however brief, is indicative of how psychoanalytic understanding can play a significant role in clinical work with asylum seekers today from a series of vantage points. To begin with, understanding the importance of initial emotional connection with someone who has suffered severe trauma, the importance of offering a space to listen and bear witness to what has been experienced is the first step towards emotional recovery as has been noted in the literature (Beritzhoff, 2021; Lijtmaer, 2017; Luci & Kahn, 2021). Secondly, consideration of the impact of trauma from a psychoanalytic perspective, which gives emphasis to bodily symptoms, dissociation, and fragmentation (Nutting, 2019; Varvin, 2017) lead to accurate diagnosis of severe clinical symptoms that have a particular meaning in the context of the traumatic experience of asylum seekers. In the case of Mr A, his presenting hallucinations without psychoanalytic intervention would most likely have been seen as a sign of psychotic disintegration and treated only with medication, preventing the exploration, understanding, and thus appropriate treatment of the symptoms.

In contrast, working from a psychoanalytic perspective enabled the analyst to consider the interpersonal dimensions that inform diagnosis – her sense of being able to make emotional contact with Mr A. – his bodily stance and eye contact led her in the direction of considering a traumatic reaction rather than a psychotic disintegration. Moreover, she considered that his hallucinatory symptoms had meaning that needed to be clarified. Keeping in mind both the cultural and internal dimensions, which have been indicated as significant (Luci & Kahn, 2021; Stitou, 2021), she carefully explored Mr A's thoughts and feelings in this regard. Her knowledge of complicated mourning, or the Ulysses syndrome, noted in the literature (Achotegui, 2019; Akhtar, 1999; Beritzhoff, 2021; Volkan, 2017), particularly with respect to guilt, and aided by her attention to transference and countertransference developments, enabled her to understand the meaning of the ghosts for Mr A. Her ability to verbalize her thoughts and communicate them to him brought evident relief for Mr A. Following a modified psychoanalytically informed technique that is typically used in work of this kind (Leuzinger-Bohleber et al., 2016; Oliner, 2014; Bohleber & Leuzinger-Bohleber, 2016), she introduced Mr A. to a way of thinking about his thoughts and feelings that allow him to understand himself and his experiences in a new and different way than before. Thus, the analyst laid a foundation for the process of symbolization and mentalization that are the ultimate goals of psychoanalytic work (Leuzinger-Bohleber, 2018; Leuzinger-Bohleber et al., 2016; Varvin, 2019).

The brevity of this intervention is in many ways poignantly limited. No sooner has an emotional connection been made than a separation ensues. However, it is a first step in the longer inner journey that will hopefully follow, leading to healing and, in time, adaptation to the reality of life in a new context.

Acknowledgements

The authors would like to thank N. Kanakis, A. Yfantis, and I. Kalyvopoulos of the NGO Doctors without Borders for their collaboration.

References

Abou-Saleh, M. T., & Chistodoulou, G. (2016, November 1). Mental health of refugees: Global perspectives. *BJPsych International*, *13*(4), 79–81.

Achotegui, J. (2019). Migrants living in very hard situations: Extreme migratory mourning (the Ulysses syndrome). *Psychoanalytic dialogues, 29*(3), 252–268.

Akhtar, S. (1999). The immigrant, the exile, and the experience of nostalgia. *Journal of Applied Psychoanalytic Studies, 1*(2), 123–130. https://doi.org/10.1023/A:1023029020496.

Amnesty International. (2020, April 3). Greece/Turkey: Asylums seekers and migrants killed and abused at borders. Retrieved from https://www.amnesty.org/en/latest/news/2020/04/greece-turkey-asylum-seekers-and-migrants-killed-and-abused-at-borders/.

Ben Farhat, J., et al. (2018). Syrian refugees in Greece: Experience with violence, mental health status and access to information during the journey and while in Greece. *BMC Medicine, 13*(16), 40.

Beritzhoff, L. C. (2021). Psychoanalysis in the meantime. *Psychoanalytic Dialogues, 31*(1), 81–99. https://doi.org/10.1080/10481885.2020.1863075

Bohleber, W., & Leuzinger-Bohleber, M. (2016). The special problem of interpretation in the treatment of traumatized patients. *Psychoanalytic Inquiry, 36,* 60–76.

Cohen, S., & Wills, T. A. (1985). Stress, social support, and the buffering hypothesis. *Psychological bulletin, 98*(2), 310.

Das, B. (2018). Mental health trauma treatment within the current Mediterranean refugee crisis. *International Journal for the Advancement of Counselling.* https://doi.org/10.1007/s10447-018-9362-y.

Doctors of the World. (2021a). *SYRIA.* Retrieved July 1, 2021, from https://doctorsoftheworld.org/project/syria/.

Doctors of the World. (2021b). *GREECE.* Retrieved July 1, 2021, from https://doctorsoftheworld.org/project/greece/.

Efstathiou, N. (2020). Nine out of 10 migrants who come to Greece are escaping violence. *Ekathimerini.* Retrieved July 1, 2021, from www.ekathimerini.com/society/249959.

Jannesari, S., Hatch, S., & Oram, S. (2020). Seeking sanctuary: Rethinking asylum and mental health. *Epidemiology and Psychiatric Sciences, 29,* E154. doi:10.1017/S2045796020000669

Jović, V. (2018). Working with traumatized refugees on the Balkan route. *International Journal of Applied Psychoanalytic Studies, 15,* 187–201. https://doi.org/10.1002/aps.1586

Kalantzakos, S. (2017). A paradox in today's Europe? Greece's response to the Syrian refugee crisis. University of the Peloponnese. *The Jean Monnet Papers on Political Economy, 15,* 1–27.

Kingsley, P. (2016). *The new odyssey: The story of Europe's refugee crisis.* London: Faber & Faber Publishing.

Ledes, R. (2019). About my film about refugees on the island of Lesvos. Testimony of Richard Ledes, author of the film No human is illegal – refugees detained on Lesvos. *Trivium: Estudos Interdisciplinares, Ano XI,* 126–128. http://dx.doi.org/10.18379/2176-4891.2019v1p.126

Leuzinger-Bohleber, M. (2018). *Finding the body in the mind: Embodied memories, trauma, and depression.* London: Routledge.

Leuzinger-Bohleber, M., & Hettich, N. (2018). What and how can psychoanalysis contribute in support of refugees? Concepts, clinical experiences and applications in the project STEP-BY-STEP, a pilot project supporting refugees in the initial reception center "Michaelisdorf"(Michaelis-village) in Darmstadt, Germany. *International Journal of Applied Psychoanalytic Studies, 15*(3), 151–173.

Leuzinger-Bohleber, M., Rickmeyer, C., Tahiri, M., Hettich, N., & Fischmann, T. (2016). What can psychoanalysis contribute to the current refugee crisis? (N. Hettich & C. Rickmeyer, Trans.). *The International Journal of Psychoanalysis, 97,* 1077–1093. https://doi.org/10.1111/1745-8315.12542

Lijtmaer, R. M. (2017). Variations on the migratory theme: Immigrants or exiles, refugee or asylees. *Psychoanalytic Review, 104,* 687–694. https://doi.org/10.1521/prev.2017.104.6.687

Luci, M., & Kahn, M. (2021). Analytic Therapy with refugees: Between silence and embodied narratives. *Psychoanalytic Inquiry, 41,* 103–114. doi:10.1080/07351690.2021.1865766.

Matziaraki, D. (2016, September 28). 4.1. Miles. *The New York Times OP-DOCS.* Retrieved from www. nytimes.com/2016/09/28/opinion/4–1-miles.html

Morina, N., Akhtar, A., Barth, J., & Schnyder, U. (2018). Psychiatric disorders in refugees and internally displaced persons after forced displacement: A systematic review. *Frontiers in Psychiatry, 9,* Article 433. doi.org/10.3389/fpsyt.2018.00433.

Nutting, T. (2019). Headaches in Moria. *British Journal of Psychotherapy International, 16,* 96–98. doi:10.1192/bji.2019.2.

Oliner, M. (2014). *Psychic reality in context.* London: Karnac Books.

Operational Data Portal. (2021). *Mediterranean situation-Greece.* Retrieved July 1, 2021, from https://data2.unhcr.org/en/situations/mediterranean/location/5179.

Orfanos, S. D. (2019). Drops of light into the darkness: Migration, immigration, and human rights. *Psychoanalytic Dialogues, 29*(3), 269–283. https://doi.org/10.10 80/10481885.2019.1614832

Poole, D. N., et al. (2018). Major depressive disorder prevalence and risk factors among Syrian asylum seekers in Greece. *BMC Public Health, 18*(1), 908.

Public Issue. (2016, January). *Erevna Gia Tis Staseis Tis Koinis Gnomis Apenandi Sto Prosfigiko Fainomeno.* (Έρευνα για τις στάσεις της κοινής γνώμης απέναντι στο προσφυγικό φαινόμενο Retrieved June 25, 2021 from. To Bima tis Kyriakis (Το Βήμα της Κυριακής).

Sperry, M., & Mull, S. (2021). Life on the line: Border stories. *Psychoanalytic Inquiry, 41*(2), 115–127. doi.org/10.1080/07351690.2021.1865769

Stitou, R. (2021). From psychic exile to geographical exile. *Psychoanalytic Psychology.* http://dx.doi.org/10.1037/pap0000333

Togashi, K., & Brothers, D. (2021). Are we all refugees? *Psychoanalytic Inquiry, 41*(2), 128–137. DOI: 10.1080/07351690.2021.1865770

Varvin, S. (2016). Psychoanalysis with the traumatized patient: Helping to survive extreme experiences and complicated loss. *International Forum of Psychoanalysis, 25*(2), 73–80. https://doi.org/10.1080/0803706X.2014.1001785

Varvin, S. (2017). Our relations to refugees: Between compassion and dehumanization. *The American Journal of Psychoanalysis, 77*(4), 359–377. https://doi.org/10.1057/s11231-017-9119-0

Varvin, S. (2019). Psychoanalysis and the situation of refugees: A human rights perspective. In P. Montagna & A. Harris (Eds.), *Psychoanalysis, law, and society* (pp. 9–26). New York: Routledge and Taylor & Francis Group.

Volkan, V. D. (2017). Psychoanalytic thoughts on the European refugee crisis and the other. *Psychoanalytic Review, 104*(6), 661–685. https://doi.org/10.1521/prev.2017.104.6.661.

World Report. (2021). *World report.* Retrieved from https://www.hrw.org/world-report/2021/country-chapters/greece.

Zarnegar, G., & Mohammadpour-Yazdi, A-R. (2021). The long winding road to liberation: The tales of two Iranian immigrants. *Psychoanalytic Inquiry, 41*(2), 91–102. DOI: 10.1080/07351690.2021.1865765

10 Is psychoanalysis of any help for refugees?

Chrysi Giannoulaki

Psychoanalysis in refugees' Lesvos – work settings

The refugee crisis has struck at the very foundation of Europe over the recent decades, and it is one of the factors determining which policies are selected by its constituent countries. Psychoanalysis is an individually based method of treatment which is mainly used "nachträglich" (differed action). Traditionally though, parallel to working in the usual psychoanalytical framework, the psychoanalytical community also aims to cultivate vigilance against racism and xenophobia and to emphasise the need for responsible participation of every citizen in the significant problems of the day, such as the major tragedies that impact every era. As part of searching for ways in which to achieve that goal, the question is also raised as to whether psychoanalysis can help respond to the refugee crisis at a hot spot, where refugees entering Greece are initially placed. In this article, I will submit a personal testimony based on my work in Moria, Lesvos, which is one of the most beleaguered first-reception areas for refugees in the Aegean Region.

I had the opportunity to go to Moria, Lesvos, as a psychoanalyst in October 2016, when the executive director of Doctors of the World (MDM), through a cooperative effort with members of the Hellenic Psychoanalytical Society to address the refugee issue, suggested I take over the supervision in Lesvos. It was to be onsite, to bolster the team of employees there, numbering around 57 in the last two months of 2016.

The team included doctors, nurses, psychologists, social workers, and administrative personnel. Indications of rifts between workers in different teams arguing with one another, irritability among carers outside of their work expressed towards the NGO's administration in Athens, expressions of complaints and hopelessness about not being able to respond to the needs of refugees were ongoing, and the constant increase in the number of workers provided no relief. It seemed that supervision could potentially help resolve this problematic situation.

Personally, I was greatly interested in what was happening in Lesvos and felt a great need to help in any way I could; I come from a family

DOI: 10.4324/9781003203223-12

of refugees myself (my grandparents were Greeks who migrated from the Asia Minor coast after World War I during the forced population exchange). I accepted the offer, though not without trepidation about what was sure to be a completely new, unfamiliar professional setting for me, moving from my private practice to a hot spot.

The working arrangement was as follows: twice a month, two two-hour group meetings were held – one on Saturday and the other on Sunday – with all staff divided into two groups. Employees were not obliged to attend and could jump from one group to another. Based on the problems that were created, I later concluded that everyone's consistent commitment to participate in one group would be preferable because it would create a stable environment that would foster more open communication of the difficult feelings experienced by participants in these traumatic conditions.

Before going, I had thought a supervisory goal could be to increase awareness of archaic defensive mechanisms among the staff and strengthen mature defensive mechanisms to support both the mental health of each member and the team's productive effectiveness. However, when I arrived in Lesvos and found myself face to face with the team of carers, I felt what it means to be the "Other" very acutely. Though I was warmly welcomed at the airport by the administrative head and the meeting with the first group took place in a well-organised space at the University of the Aegean, the coldness in the faces of carers when I entered the room warned me of what would be a harsh rejection: what would I, as a psychoanalyst with a comfortable office in Athens, have to offer these people tormented by insomnia and desperation who pulled dead children from the sea, who could not play with their own children because of the guilt they felt, who did not know how to deal with illnesses, the mourning and anger of the refugees, who did not even know if they would still have a job after the few months of their contract were up? They directed these questions at me immediately, accompanied by a terse final refusal: "We don't need help from a supervisor, tell the main office. We need translators and a psychiatrist for the refugees!"

I felt useless, hopeless, and alone. Was it perhaps arrogant of me to go? A psychoanalyst at a hot spot! What did I know about conditions of war? Fortunately, my psychoanalytical thinking, used to violent rejections even on an individual level, was helpful to me: perhaps I felt as they did? Perhaps they made me feel what they were unable to tell me?

I therefore decided to respond by accepting that I could not offer everything they needed, but to persist in my desire to lend a hand in their struggle and their pain. I told them I believe that by understanding what we feel and talking about our reactions as freely as possible, we could pave a small part of the road for the refugees and for our own. I told them I understood their anger – they are not alone in reacting this way in similar conditions. At all refugee camps, anger and detachment are the main defences erected for survival, not just for refugees but for carers as well.

And so the ice began to thaw a little at that meeting. First, they asked me to fill the gap in appropriate psychiatric care. Many refugees were arriving in Lesvos daily after months-long journeys. The long-term stay of refugees at the camp increased the need to address the psychological problems that inevitably arose once survival needs were met and physical illnesses were treated. As one might expect, particularly acute posttraumatic syndromes and a variety of anxiety disorders and psychotic disorganisations in vulnerable patients created the need for psychiatric diagnosis and medication. There was only one psychiatric clinic on the entire island, at the Lesvos hospital, and just one psychiatrist, who naturally could not see all those refugees needing treatment.

I accepted their proposal. Abandoning the security of my "tidy" professional identity, as a team supervisor at the university campus on the island and my transfer to the chaos of Moria made me less of an "Other" and more one of them. In turn, I would also experience the desperation of people who waited for me in an endless queue outside the makeshift shack, the worry over finding an interpreter, to try to understand in ten minutes what was happening and how I could help, and then rushing to get on the plane at the last minute, full of guilt about how little I had contributed but also eager to return. There is beauty in human diversity and, moreover, to be part of a human tragedy may capture your inner life!

In the supervisory groups, in Lesvos, we talked about ourselves and about the refugees. We discovered that the refugees are not just nice people who will accept our help with gratitude so we can go home feeling good that we provided something that made a difference. These are deeply traumatised people, which makes them angry, irritable, frustrated, often being not able to speak but expressing their inner disaster in physical pain. They are demanding; they have regressed and demand some kind of compensation for all they have been through – often, they expect to find themselves in paradise.

Moreover, they are people who often suffer from a pathology that contributed to their leaving their country and which must be diagnosed and treated. Many of them could not cope with what had happened to them and resorted to escape in search of an idealised parent who would solve their problems. That is why they believed the smugglers who promised them that, in Lesvos, they would be put on a bus and sent to Germany (one mother got into a boat leaving her baby behind with another woman to bring along on the next, better boat, which never came). Or they place their trust in the pimp who promises them easy money through prostitution or drugs. They are people who, because they feel guilty about those they left behind, unconsciously seek punishment and, thus, in a negative therapeutic response, reject the help they are being given. They have been betrayed many times, and while they demand everything, they do not believe in nor cooperate on anything.

Last but not least, they are people who do not speak the same language as we do. Communication is mediated by an interpreter, with all that entails for a modern Tower of Babel, which further discourages them from wanting to communicate.

In the supervisory groups, discussions over what homeland means for each of us, what home means, and the nostalgia each one feels for his country created a warmer atmosphere which threw light on the discussion about what so many European volunteers coming to Lesvos from the start of the refugee crisis were looking for: the search for the refugee within themselves, outside of the routine of everyday life, an opportunity for psychological maturity and enrichment.

There was a period of a few months when hopes for creating stability and security were fulfilled. But political changes in how NGOs operate soon threw the team back into a state of hopelessness and anger. The older refugees were trapped on the island, while the newer arrivals were leaving for Athens, benefiting from new regulations. The NGOs argued among themselves over the vulnerability verifications that would allow some refugees to travel to Athens. The sense of injustice and helplessness prevailed.

Gradually, many of the carers requested individual sessions with me. I recognised signs of burnout in most of them: grief, diminished emotional response, flashbacks to the things they heard from refugees in their interactions, insomnia, and alcohol abuse as a response to anxiety were apparent in most and led them to break off relationships in their personal life or in many cases feel the impact on their marriage. We talked about how they had remained in traumatic conditions for a very long time, caring for very traumatised people. We discussed the need for breaks when someone takes on such a difficult task. Some of the carers found meeting with me helped them to overcome their guilt to leave the island. I met with some of them later in Athens. At some point, I noticed that I was also beginning to have trouble sleeping, something that I had never experienced in this way in my life. My work in Athens seemed meaningless, and I became short-tempered with friends when we disagreed. I was taken by surprise. So I recognised that I was also exhausted and had to do what I was advising others to do: pass on the baton and continue my work with the refugees in Athens. I hope this article will be part of what I pray to pass on.

In summary, my work in Lesvos took place on four levels:

- The first was supervising the team, the initial reason for my being hired.
- The second was my personal work with refugees.
- The third was my personal work with carers.
- The fourth was my internal work on myself every minute that I was in Lesvos.

I will attempt to provide an example for each one of these areas.

A) Team supervision

As already mentioned, the carers' work was particularly demanding and largely impossible. They were required to operate in an organised manner in a completely chaotic setting and to meet the medical needs of a deeply traumatised population in conditions which only prolong their traumatisation and which act as a trauma in the "here and now."

Here are a few examples. A nurse named Christos said tensely that he realised from the odour there was sepsis resulting from frostbite in a newly arrived refugee who had not sought help because he was so exhausted from the journey; he could not even think about his foot. Christos was taking him to Doctors of the World, who were in Moria at that time, and he was able to begin treatment aimed at not amputating the whole foot, but just some toes that could not be saved. I observed for myself one of the daily dressing changes performed by the nurse even when he was not on duty so that the care of this refugee would not be overlooked in the oncoming wave of new arrivals. In the midst of so many more serious needs of the refugees, Christos did not dare to complain about the incessant workload for fear that he would betray his ideals.

The discussion helped others become aware of the silence they observed about major daily incidents that angered them in their work, worried that they would become a burden, and turned it against themselves and felt guilty about their inability to respond on a practically 24-hour basis to all the problems that arose. We discovered that the heroic nature of rescuing refugees' lives that includes concealing the angry responses that form internally leads to the dissociation not only from part of the carers' own psyche, but also from the local community. Christos would get furious with any Lesvos resident who complained about the change in their way of life because of the refugees and who resorted to using racist expressions against them. In so doing, however, he was unable to help the locals understand their xenophobic and racist responses which, on the other hand, could be expected to arise when the arrival of so many newcomers with a different language, religions, manner of dress, appearance, and so on threated to disrupt their large-group identity as Greek, orthodox, inhabitants of Lesvos!

A reminder of the complexity of the issue from a psychoanalytical perspective was particularly constructive, as the excellent cooperation of all involved is essential to helping refugees better adapt so that, for example, their children can be more readily accepted at the playground alongside the local children.

We also talked about the xenophobia and racism which lie dormant in each of us, and which emerge even with the slightest stimuli, upsetting the image one might have of the distressed refugee he wants to help. Unaccompanied teens who played loud music or self-harmed were often subjected to rejection by staff, who forcefully and without any empathy demanded they be removed from the camp. Taking part in this campaign to have them removed were not just careers but also many of the other refugees who lived in the same facility and were often from the same country.

In the introduction to the book *Immigrants and Refugees. Trauma, Perennial Mourning, Prejudice and Border Psychology* (2017), Volkan refers to a similar incident relayed by a well-known German psychoanalyst who was overcome by an intense desire to combat racism and provide asylum to refugees. While the psychoanalyst was resting in a train compartment, a preadolescent child from Syria came in looking for somewhere to charge an iPhone he had with him. The psychoanalyst, sensitive as he was to identifying his internal responses, realised this image of the child with the expensive phone in his hand was in stark contrast with the image of a subject who is suffering and whom he wants to help. The experienced therapist was consciously aware of the annoyance that this contrast caused him internally, and he soon escaped. Nevertheless, Volkan quite correctly brings it up, believing that we can learn much from this momentary response. I told the group about the incident to encourage some thought on such a difficult issue.

Finally, we often referred to the strong ties among the team members and the sense of humour of many employees that lightened the burden of such a difficult mission. When emotions become unbearable, someone would ask them to come up with a funny story to make us laugh.

At the end of group, there would often be a reference to the natural beauty of Lesvos. Employees who were from Lesvos would talk about their fields and agricultural chores, creating an embrace from nature and a promise of returning to peace and life.

B) *Working with refugees*

One important point which is not usually stressed enough is that, aside from being deeply traumatised, refugees are people who have managed to survive in exceedingly adverse conditions, where many others failed. Naturally, this engenders in them a deep sense of guilt which, along with the ongoing trauma of being treated as undesirables, does not allow them to acknowledge feelings such as pride in the fact they succeeded or joy about being alive or even to feel hope for the future. The recognition of such feelings and of what they achieved and continue to achieve is part of the recognition of their human condition and their need to retain their dignity amidst such difficult circumstances. A reminder of this protects from attempting to self-harm and from reacting violently towards others.

Here is an example: X. came to the clinic with insomnia, irritability, anxiety, and panic attacks. I gave him anti-anxiety medication to calm him and help him sleep and told him to come back the following week. At our second meeting, X. was in a terrible state: he looks at the floor, cries, says he will kill himself, that he cannot take any more, that here is worse than being in prison, that he is afraid of the barbed wire he sees around him and that it reminds him of prison in Iran. He talked so loudly that the interpreter seemed to reach his limit and said he cannot interpret if the beneficiary speaks so fast and so intensely. I feared that, with the interpreter mentally giving up, I would not be able to do anything. Once again, I felt alone. To calm myself and think, I turned my attention to the children who were yelling outside, in the camp. I remembered then that the psychologist who referred X. to me wrote that he had a son in Iran. I told the interpreter, "[T]ell him that I know he has a son. Ask him if he has contacted him." On hearing this, the beneficiary stopped being withdrawn; he looked at me and said, "Yes, I have a son, but I can't contact him because I'm afraid I will put him and my wife in danger and I'm very worried. I am in a panic."

He told me his story, at least the story that he could tell a doctor initially. X. is an Arab (which means he is Sunni; 95% of Arabs are Sunnis) from Iran (where they are Shiites). In Iran, they captured his father in the street during a random raid because he did not respond appropriately to questions – perhaps due to the onset of dementia – so he was condemned to death. He was hung in prison with X. present. X. had also been imprisoned and in fact had a finger cut off for making a forbidden gesture with his hand. When his brother was also imprisoned, X. decided to abandon the country, leaving behind in Iran his 13/14-year-old son and his wife.

I told the interpreter to translate:

> [T]ell him that I will not give him more drugs – the medicine is his desire to help his son and wife to be safe. He made an awfully long journey to be here and save himself, but also his loved ones in the future. If he kills himself, he will be free of anxiety and guilt, but he won't be helping anyone.

The beneficiary looked me in the eyes and smiled faintly and tiredly. He nodded his head and said, "Yes. It was an exceedingly difficult journey." The next time he waited for me outside the camp and greeted me with a smile. He did not come to the clinic.

C) Working with carers

Those working in the refugee first-reception field are people with a particularly marked a) desire to help b) ability to derive joy from this and c) ability to give "meaning" to their work when they help fellow human beings in need.

Much like the refugees who need the recognition of their bravery and love for those they left behind, carers also need recognition for the characteristics mentioned above. Acceptance of their positive traits helps them to process their guilt over their finite capacity to respond and to channel their desire to help into acquiring additional "thinking tools."

In individual sessions, starting from the intercultural perspective, we often discussed each person's personal journey from their own place of origin to Lesvos. As they felt safer than in the group, we discovered that a significant and frequently recurring aspect of an unseen racism disguised as pity was the rejection not of the refugees themselves – that would easily be condemned by the conscience – but of what the refugees bring with them, such as their diversity. In this way, their mental reality was frequently contradicted. After interpreting the conversion of the therapeutic stance to humanism as a defensive mechanism against guilt, depending on the case, I stressed their desire to strengthen their identity. For example, in our individual sessions, I urged Christos to continue his studies at nursing school in Athens. Another example: M. experienced a brief psychotic break. I referred him to a colleague I knew, supporting his desire to recover and continue his work. He contacted me later to thank me and to tell me that he would now be more sensitive to people who presented with similar problems and that, for the time being, he would work in calmer conditions at homeless shelters in Athens.

It became even clearer to me that, to care for refugees, you must first take care of their carers. We determined that this revelation is particularly important to addressing the refugee issue. We organised a two-day symposium on this topic in Athens, where several people working in Lesvos at the time spoke.

D) *An everyday experience – children's play*

Unaccompanied minors live in shipping containers in an enclosed space in front of the first-reception area. On Sundays, when I went to the camp to see refugee patients, the children were usually playing in front of the gate, which kept the space enclosed. One Sunday, as I was leaving hurriedly to catch the flight to Athens, I found the gate closed, and six to seven kids aged five to eight outside shouting "ID! ID!" For a few seconds, I did not understand what was happening and felt a wave of fear disproportionate to both my position and my age before this small mob of tiny guards keeping me prisoner in the camp, sealing the gate with a piece of string from a toy.

To calm myself, I automatically resorted to Freud's grandson's Fort/Da, which transported me to another space – the space of thought – and took me away from the place of violence in which I found myself.

Meanwhile, a guard intervened, the door was opened, and I managed to make the flight. Even though it came from children, even though it was a game, I kept hearing the voices calling out, "ID no good! No good ID!" over the next few days, and I remember the sparks of fury in the eyes of the young refugees, alongside the excited joy at playing a child's game. I detected a miniature posttraumatic disorder in myself and was surprised once again by the intensity of traumatic transference.

Conclusion

Concern over whether and in what manner the psychoanalytic community can contribute to responding to the major disasters of our times, including the refugee issue, has been growing within the International Psychoanalytical Association. Through my experience, I conclude that psychoanalytical thought could be a significant contributor to the endeavour to care for both the refugees themselves and for their carers. Psychoanalytical literature has studied trauma and its intergenerational transfer extensively and could convey important aspects of the need for treatment in as timely a manner as possible. The psychodynamic supervision proved beneficial for the proper function of each worker, so that each beneficiary could receive the best care possible from them. But it also protected workers from the risk of burnout and their own traumatic disorder resulting from ongoing exposure to the intensely traumatic experiences of the beneficiaries.

Naturally, there is a need for further research into whether and how psychoanalysis could be of help at a hot spot that would provide data to investigate this question further.

Reference

Volkan, D. V. (2017). *Immigrants and refugees. Trauma, perennial mourning, prejudice and border psychology*. London: Karnac Books.

11 Schizoid mechanisms in posttraumatic states

Vladimir Jović

Introduction and background

Prolonged wars in Iraq and Syria, continuous armed conflict in Afghanistan, combined with extremely difficult life and economic uncertainties from Central Asia to sub-Saharan Africa resulted in huge waves of refugees[1] passing through the "Balkan route" to Europe, which peaked in 2015 (Jović, 2018). Their reception in Europe by political elites was at best ambivalent – welcoming attitudes were very scarce. Instead, they were used or abused "by a noisy right wing movement" (Varvin, 2017), which perpetuated narratives of dangerous foreigners, fundamentalists, European culture suddenly being threatened, and so on. Of course, this was also followed by many empathic responses, both at the level of some European governments and the public in some countries which probably still keep alive collective traumas of exile (ibid.).

More important is that the huge percentage of refugees were severely traumatised in their countries of origin, either as civilians exposed to direct combat such as bombardment of large urban areas, ethnic cleansing and forcible expulsion, direct atrocities – massive killings, torture and rape, often used as a weapon of war. From many individual reports it became apparent that these armed conflicts have taken the form of "new wars," which do not involve states in conflict and battles between armies, but instead involve many different fighting factions and most usually employ violence against civilians (Kaldor, 2013). In that context, multiple, prolonged, and diverse traumatic experiences are very frequent.

Adding to all of this, we have numerous reports about abuse and torture during exile, including within European countries (Jović, 2017, 2018, 2021). In March 2016, the so-called Balkan route was closed, which in reality meant employing police, border police, and army together with barbwired fences and other physical obstacles to prevent refugees from entering countries, chasing and arresting them beyond the border only to be expelled (pushed back) across the border that they just crossed. These "group pushbacks" are followed by physical violence, including systematic beatings, use of pepper spray, attacks by police dogs, among other

DOI: 10.4324/9781003203223-13

forms, and they should be regarded as a torture, as defined by the 1987 UN Convention against Torture. While difficult to comprehend by any human standards, these acts of violence do have their inner "logic" as they represent a "deterrent torture": "its aim is to discourage or encourage certain activities on the part of the victim or other people, or perhaps both" ((Tindale, 1996), pp. 350–351). As far as we know, this is happening all over the region in an apparently organised political coordination by most Balkan countries and with at least silent support from the European Union: "The EU's institutions and the member states . . . have chosen to largely ignore [the human rights violations (HRV) connected with the closure of the Balkan route, and] this ignorance in practice amounts to a tacit agreement" (Weber, 2017).

For mental health professionals of my generation, this is the second time that we are faced with huge numbers of severely traumatised individuals, as we already have had waves of refugees during wars in ex-Yugoslavia in 1990s, some of whom were severely traumatised and tortured (Špirić et al., 2004). Comparisons and lessons learned are hard to avoid telling (Jović, 2021). And again, we have a new generation of professionals confronted with the complexity of psychological trauma and posttraumatic states who are trying to comprehend the suffering of others and develop techniques to provide effective support and treatment. They bring in, either in consultation or in supervision, different theories, explicit or implicit, about the psychological trauma, pathogenic mechanisms, and therapeutic skills that they have acquired in different settings. Over time it became compelling to try to elucidate the many complex psychoanalytical theories of trauma and contrast them with the other concepts, which were mainly relying on the prevailing biomedical concept of posttraumatic stress disorder (PTSD).

Posttraumatic syndrome

At the time when wars in the former Yugoslavia erupted, we already had PTSD as a nosological entity that allowed mental health professionals to claim that the person is suffering due to experience related to war (and other traumas as well); to decrease stigma related to psychiatric treatment; and to cover costs of treatment and rehabilitation, sometimes even compensation – unless politics come into play (Opačić et al., 2006).

In the clinic, we could see a lot of what has been included in the DSM-III-R criteria (American Psychiatric Association, 1987): refugees were complaining about insomnia, nightmares, and repetitive dreaming about war; they would be aroused if someone talked about war or if something reminded them about it (men in uniforms, like postmen, trenches for electrical cables which resembled war trenches), they would avoid talking about their experiences (watching news on TV or movies with war themes) or would become agitated and have outbursts of anger if some-one talked about war. Many described a lack of interest in pleasurable activities or detachment from others ("I take my grandson in my arms as if I hold a chair"), hypervigilance and startle response, but there was much, much more.

There was a myriad of other mental symptoms or disorders, such as many forms of anxiety; panic attacks; structured agoraphobia; depressive states from stupor to severe depression with psychotic symptoms; hal-lucinatory states sometimes in the form of "bizarre objects" (Jović, 2002) or auditory hallucinations which a person understood as memory (of real voices of the enemy threatening them); many cases of severe substance abuse, sometimes combined with gambling; violent criminal activities (usually among adolescents); self-harm; and risk-taking behaviour, from reckless driving to fighting in bars. There was guilt – overwhelming, unbearable, often denied and then expressed in outbursts of desperation, self-harm, and intoxications.[2] Much less common were dissociative states, more often described by family members than by patients. And there was pain: chronic, intense, usually located in one or a couple of body parts, headaches, pain in the chest, lower back, hands, wrists; medicines would help just for a short period of time. Following the logic of DSM, all these symptoms would be transformed into disorders and enlisted as "comor-bidity," which might be an artefact stemming from a never-made-explicit rule that the same symptom could not appear in criteria for more than one disorder (Maj, 2005).

Then there were physical illnesses which could be related to traumatic experiences: severe and treatment-resistant hypertension, endocrinologic and metabolic disturbances – for example, insulin resistance syndrome, with consequential diabetes and cardiovascular disorders – rapid ageing, and increased morbidity and mortality (Špirić, 2008). We will probably need more systematic research on refugee families which will try to com-prehensibly assess both mental and physical disorders and try to bridge the ever-increasing gap between somatic medicine and the psychology of stress.

And then there is this huge area which we cannot readily label as symp-toms, but nevertheless, these perceptions and complaints are an expres-sion of anguish and strain: astonishment with the bizarreness of war; with the pure evil that happened before their eyes; betrayal and corruption; collapse of laws, morale, and civilisation; disillusionment with politics, demagogy, and ideology, which set all this destruction into motion; feel-ings of being sacrificed while others got away and continued their lives; transformation of close friends and neighbours, sometime schoolmates, into bitter enemies who would kill or torture; incapacities of military officers and politicians; foolishness and recklessness of others in critical moments; sheer luck or lack of it in plain death or survival; and so on. All these stories could be understood as shock after witnessing a collapse of social order and meaning, loss of sense of a safe interpersonal field, and an overpowering destruction of dehumanisation.

The very first descriptions of "Post-Vietnam Syndrome" by Chaim Shatan, (Shatan, 1972) closely related to the narratives of my clients. Shatan enlists "guilt feelings for those killed and maimed on both sides," "they have been scapegoats . . . they feel deceived, used and betrayed," "rage [because of] the awareness of being duped and manipulated," and dehumanisation during basic training and in the warzone: "Every time you acted human, you got screwed" (Shatan, 1973, p. 647). In fact, we can say that all these complaints are related to the interpersonal/social sphere (Rosenbaum et al., 2020).

There are written histories of how Chatan's original Post-Vietnam Syndrome became PTSD (Shephard, 2001; Young, 1995), with help from Mardi J. Horowitz who used the information processing model to define three clusters of symptoms – intrusion, avoidance, and hyperarousal (Rosenbaum et al., 2020). Thus, the implicit pathogenetic mechanism of PTSD became inadequate processing of traumatic memory, which "jumps up" into the mind in a form of intrusive re-experiencing and needs to be avoided as it creates an unpleasant hyperarousal. Memory of traumatic events was described as unchanged by any mental processes and imagined like an exact "recording," although we know that memory is not stored in a recording camera fashion. Even during the storage there is a process of selection and recreation or reconstruction during which "we add on feelings, beliefs, or even knowledge we obtained after the experience. In other words, we bias our memories of the past by attributing to them emotions or knowledge we acquired after the event" (Schacter, quoted in: (Bohleber, 2007)). In the same manner, traumatic dreams became "replicative dreams," "an exact replay ('replication') of the original event" (Schreuder et al., 1998) – which designates that they are not dreams proper, mental materials changed by the dream work, but explicit memory of the event that happened in reality. The path for "memory wars" was opened and is still not closed (Patihis et al., 2013). In practical terms, mainstream treatment for PTSD became "trauma-focused psychotherapies" (Rosenbaum et al., 2020).

Posttraumatic mental states

While descriptive psychopathology takes segments of subject's behaviour (action and narrations) as basic units of its analysis, biological psychiatry is focused on changes in structure and functions of the brain. In psychoanalysis, the objects of analysis are unconscious phantasies, which we reach through free associations, analysis of dreams and material stemming from transference/countertransference phenomena.

It is worth remembering that "psychoanalysis began as a theory of trauma" (Bohleber, 2007); after abandoning what will later be called "seduction theory," Freud developed a number of concepts which will aim to explain a "psychic reality." Paradoxically, psychoanalysis from its start was focused on childhood (traumatic) memories and many valuable, more complementary than contradictory, concepts were developed (Baranger et al., 1988). At the same time "trauma theory long remained a desideratum of analytic research [and] did not have the status in psychoanalysis that it should in fact have commanded" [as one of the reasons being that] "[m]ost analysts directed their attention more or less exclusively to the inner world and to the question of the influence of unconscious phantasies on perceptions and the shaping of internal object relationships" (Bohleber, 2007, p. 330).

If we try to be less critical, maybe it is more proper to say that we needed time to have some other, extremely important concepts to be developed, especially those that explain our mental processes as a continuous interaction with external objects (projection and projective identification, container/contained, transitional object and transitional space) and processes that explain functioning and development of mental apparatus (Bion's theory of thinking, alpha function, and so on, as well as the concept of symbolisation and mentalisation, to name just a few). This allows us to see the dynamics of fragmentation and integration in posttraumatic personality, splitting of parts of the experience that are unbearable, but also splitting of psychic functions that are able to perceive, remember, and mentalise that experience.

> The human mind has the power to isolate experiences that are painful to it or actively attempt to isolate itself from these. [Work of Freud, Klein, Bion, and Meltzer led to understanding that] two or more parts of the self can be split in the mental world and go on to living lives that are concomitant and isolated, functioning according to their own mental logic and differing among themselves.
>
> (da Rocha Barros, 2009, p. xvii)

A couple more statements from this short overview are worth quoting here:

> Klein also introduces the idea that a part split off from the personality, ejected outwards, can later be reincorporated. Bion takes a step further, suggesting that not only parts of the self can be split, but also mental functions. The more immediate consequence of mental splitting is the impoverishment of mental life. When a patient separates from a painful and unbearable emotion, he is also splitting from the part of the self capable of having that emotion. This impoverishment occurs in

various manners. The person loses a sense of continuity of his mental life so that his capacity to hold himself responsible for his feelings and actions is diminished, and thus his capacity to interfere in his destiny is brutally affected. On splitting due to loss of links between emotional experiences, the capacity for symbolizing and the possibility of construction of mental representations is sensibly hindered.

(ibid. p. xviii)

I believe that this is a crucial mechanism which can explain acute as well as chronic disabling posttraumatic states, like in individuals who survived torture, and I will try to support it with short clinical vignettes.

We can now conceive of the consequences of psychological trauma as a result of a schizoid process, governed by a splitting of more or less large "chunks" of mental apparatus and damage being done by this process. As splitting is a result of an unbearable experience, we assume that the first step would be anxiety about such an intensity (hence, the concept of "stimulus barrier") that can destroy the protective shield – that is, safety system developed in more or less favourable psychosexual development, which is in essence equal to the "unbinding" of instincts. Unleashed death instinct, released of its neutralising counterpart – good, soothing, nurturing force developed through the introjection of a relationship with (a good enough) primary object cannot be perceived in a mentalised way, but is experienced as "psychotic anxiety," "annihilation anxiety," or "nameless dread" (to name just a few of the many concepts). This first step, overwhelming anxiety and unbinding, I described earlier (Jović, 2018), and I would like to focus on splitting and evacuative projective identification, which depletes the personality and is probably the main mechanism in posttraumatic states. In that sense, we go from "syndrome" or a list of behavioural indicators, towards an understanding of the dynamics of a pathological mental state, which is induced by overwhelming (thus – "traumatic") anxieties as a reaction to an external event.

As anxiety cannot be mentalised, fragments of the self are split off and evacuated, probably in more than one way and form. It seems that in chronic cases damage becomes a kind of pathological position (in Steiner's sense of the term), which impedes full integration, through mourning and achievement of a depressive position. But at the same time, it does not (often) lead to full (psychotic) disintegration. What is left is a kind of psychological "balancing" – avoiding remembering and probably continuous and repetitive evacuation, which leaves a person in a kind of frozen state and in a narrow corridor where psychological functioning is possible, with restricted affect and damaged affective modulation; impoverished interpersonal relationships; loss of psychological functions that are needed for integration; fragility and sensitivity that necessitates supportive, containing, and soothing relationships; medicines or drugs, or evacuative repetitive actions.

Case A. A woman, who was in her forties and imprisoned and tortured in a concentration camp in Bosnia for ten months, eventually reunited with her family and lived in Belgrade at the time when I met her. She had full support from her husband and children and many friends, but she could not work, could not socialise, and most of the time, she would spend in a room either in a numb and frozen state or in attacks of desperation. Rare activities were silent walks with her husband. When she came to my office, she was calm; she said that she did not want any psychotherapy, but it was very important for her to know she could come to me for help if she "collapses" (mentally). What was worrying her and what she anticipated as a danger was an invitation to appear as a witness in front of the International Criminal Tribunal for the former Yugoslavia (ICTY). Though it would be organised over a video link, for her, being in contact with this horrific experience signalled a psychological catastrophe, which eventually happened – a couple of months after, she came to me in a complete state of desperation, crying, almost screaming, as the session with ICTY had been scheduled. For me, it was visible that what created a crisis was not a memory but *being in a mental state* which was the same as the concentration camp–related mental state (I believe that this is an indicator of impaired symbolisation due to massive projective identification and symbolic equation). This state had been evacuated and kept at a distance as much as possible, with considerable cost of impoverished psychic life and in constant threat of reappearance in the mind.

Bollas developed a phrase "fascist state of mind," explaining the dynamics behind (not only fascist) ideology. Among many valuable observations, I found most important the idea that the achievement of such a cruel state of mind has been accomplished by splitting and "killing" off human parts. The subject, as composed of varied parts of the self, achieves its complexity through the integration of these parts, which Bollas compares to a "parliamentary order with instincts, memories, needs, anxieties, and object responses" (Bollas, 1992, p. 197). But under the strain (anxiety), parts of the self are projected onto other objects, and this operation can denude a person from more complex, empathic, and understanding human parts: "humanity is presumably represented or representable by the presence of different capacities of the self (such as empathy, forgiveness, and reparation) which had been squeezed out of the self" (ibid. p. 198). I will not go any further into this very rich text, but simply repeat (Jović, 2021) that this mechanism of "dehumanisation" is in essence a schizoid process of evacuating empathic, human parts of the self in order to avoid guilt and unbearable anxiety. Dehumanisation is also a mechanism of preparation for war, either through demonising the enemy through war propaganda or as a part of soldiers' training (drill), which in essence aims to remove all personal characteristics and individuality and create a successful soldier, which is the same as creating an efficient killer – a person whose human capacities have been taken away, so he can dehumanise the enemy and kill him. I have seen it with many soldiers who develop severe psychic crises not at the front line but upon the return to safety (so-called delayed onset PTSD), when these empathic human parts will require reintegration. I believe that this was described by Chatan as well when he spoke about the "grief of soldiers" and treatment as "re-humanisation."

Case B. Just near the end of the war in Bosnia, I received a young man who spent several years at the front line, fighting in some kind of special units and who described his behaviour, which in military terms would be considered as acts of epic heroism, but in fact were unbelievable cruel. He did not tell me those things as a way of praising his courage and skills, but instead, he was describing a horror of unimaginable intensity that he survived. At the very entrance to my office, he exclaimed: "Doctor, whatever you ask, do not ask if I feel guilt!" The main reason for him asking for help was a state of complete desperation as his first child had just been born. He spoke about this as a horrible mistake to have let this thing happen. For me, it was obvious that the birth of his child created a crisis, as his human, empathic parts would be needed in his new life, but at the same time, this would create a depressive collapse over guilt and remorse.

Case C. A young man, 17 years old, left Afghanistan some ten months before I met him, after his family was annihilated while he was away from the village. He complained about headaches, pain in other parts of the body, lack of sleep, and thoughts about suicide; his case manager described outbursts of anger. As I described this case earlier (Jović, 2018), I will focus on one particular set of phenomena. He spoke about "ghosts" that appeared during the night, behind him (he showed me how he turns his head to check what is behind him), but also spoke about his fears of walking through some parts of Belgrade where he expected to meet other people from Afghanistan (it was true that there was some violence with lethal assaults within that group). When these aggressive outbursts happened during our sessions, it became obvious that they were the evacuation of unbearable feelings. Only after a few more sessions did he tell me that he was unaware of the fate of his two younger brothers and a sister, and a first outcry of sadness overwhelmed him. It seems that these split off parts, either in a non-incarnated form (as "ghosts") or as persecutory objects are easily observed in acute cases. Another case might illustrate that.

Case D (discussed in group supervision, presented in detail in: (Rosenbaum et al., 2020)). An 18-year-old refugee from the Middle East who had an extremely hard life over the past couple of years was referred to counselling by a social worker, though he did not have any complaints, and his overall attitude was one of the "survivors," the "resilient man." What was creating confusion in the group was the fact that although he had a series of extremely traumatic experiences, he did not apparently express any "posttraumatic symptoms." It was obvious that these experiences did not *become traumatic* for him yet (hence the concept of *Nachträglichkeit*). But he used to offer narratives which were instructive about the intensity of his projections. He decided to stay in Serbia though "you have no cuisine, no music, no culture, and no history as old as in the Arab world." But other countries were no good anymore:

> And yet, to go to Germany, which is full of Afghans, who spoil the reputation of refugees because they act like animals, who do not know what soap is and are so primitive and ungrateful, they destroy everything that is afforded to them.

Instead, he filled in sessions (with a female therapist) with stories of women and girls trying to seduce him, which he resisted in fear. It resembled Rosenfeld's description, which Bollas (1992) quoted in the paper on fascist state of mind, of destructive narcissism as an organised gang which prevents any part of the self from libidinal attachment. Depressive collapse eventually came not too many weeks after, when he learned that his younger brother ended up in the same ordeal as he previously did. That opened up a possibility not only to empathise with his brother but also with his own story of trauma, suffering, and pain.

In a last, very brief case (**case E**), I would like to illustrate how psychological functions could be evacuated, in this case, a function of knowing (Laub & Auerhahn, 1993), of comprehending traumatic experience. A woman at the end of her professional career was preparing to leave Belgrade and travel back to her country of origin. She came asking for help due to severe, persistent insomnia, for which she could not find a cure (medicines, hypnotherapy). For many sessions she would just complain about it in a desperate way, completely helpless and without hope. Eventually, she started to pace in front of me, through the office in a repetitive manner. It took us both some time until we connected it to the following story: some 40 years ago, she was imprisoned with a couple of friends (no one else survived) because of political activities, but eventually she was released because of the social influence of her family. She said something like this: "I *do not know* how many days and nights I spent in the cell, I *do not know* was I tortured, and I *do not know* if I was raped." It was interesting that even while confirming what kind of trauma she survived, she still denied to herself (and to me) a knowledge of it.

Conclusion

Understanding methodological differences behind differing psychopathological conceptualisations of posttraumatic reactions can probably ease our confusion about their protean nature. Expression of posttraumatic suffering is not a single set of symptoms nor a simple one. I tried to explain that through understanding schizoid mechanisms, splitting and projective identification as well as reintegration via mourning, we can grasp much wider spectrums of expressions and modify our technique that should be aimed at reintegrating individuals at the proper time and with the best possible support.

Notes

1 As always, I do not intend here to make a difference between refugee, migrant, or asylum seeker, as all of those are legal categories, and the focus of this paper is on the psychological experience of displacement, migration, trauma and abuse. Varvin notes how all these different terms are used with political and ideological implications and are used differently in media as well (Varvin, 2017).
2 In the original description in DSM-III in 1980, guilt was included in criteria for PTSD: "guilt about surviving when others have not, or about behaviour required for survival" (American Psychiatric Association, 1980, p. 238), but then it was excluded in DSM-III-R.

References

American Psychiatric Association. (1980). *Diagnostic and statistical manual of mental disorders* (3rd ed.). Washington, DC: American Psychiatric Association.

American Psychiatric Association. (1987). *Diagnostic and statistical manual of mental disorders* (3rd ed., Rev.). Washington, DC: American Psychiatric Association.

Baranger, M., Baranger, W., & Mom, J. M. (1988). The infantile psychic trauma from us to Freud: Pure trauma, retroactivity and reconstruction. *The International Journal of Psycho-Analysis, 69*, 113.

Bohleber, W. (2007). Remembrance, trauma and collective memory: The battle for memory in psychoanalysis. *The International Journal of Psychoanalysis, 88*(2), 329–352.

Bollas, C. (1992). The fascist state of mind. In *Being a character; psychoanalysis and self experience* (pp. 193–217). London: Routledge.

da Rocha Barros, E. M. (2009). Foreword. In T. Bokanowski & S. Lewkowicz (Eds.), *On Freud's "splitting of the ego in the process of defence"* (pp. xv–xx). London: Karnac Books.

Jović, V. (2002). Trauma and the other. In S. Varvin & T. Štajner Popović (Eds.), *Upheaval: Psychoanalytical perspectives on trauma* (pp. 81–100). Belgrade: International Aid Network.

Jović, V. (2017). Kriegstrauma, migration und ihre konsequenzen. In M. Leuzinger-Bohleber, U. Bahrke, S. Hau, T. Fischmann, & S. Arnold (Eds.), *Flucht, migration und trauma: Die Folgen für die nächste Generation* (pp. 175–198). Göttingen: Vandenhoeck & Ruprecht GmbH & Co.

Jović, V. (2018). Working with traumatized refugees on the Balkan route. *International Journal of Applied Psychoanalytic Studies*, 187–201.

Jović, V. (2021). Refugees, torture and dehumanization. In D. Bughra (Ed.), *Oxford textbook of migrant psychiatry* (pp. 351–358). Oxford: Oxford University Press.

Kaldor, M. (2013). *New and old wars: Organised violence in a global era*. New Jersey: John Wiley & Sons.

Laub, D., & Auerhahn C. N. (1993). Knowing and not knowing massive psychic trauma: Forms of traumatic memory. *International Journal of Psycho-Analysis, 74*, 287–302.

Maj, M. (2005). 'Psychiatric comorbidity': An artefact of current diagnostic systems? *The British Journal of Psychiatry, 186*(3), 182–184.

Opačić, G., Jović, V., Radović, B., & Knežević, G. (2006). *Redress in action: Consequences of forcible mobilization of refugees in 1995.* Belgrade: International Aid Network.

Patihis, L., Ho, L. Y., Tingen, I. W., Lilienfeld, S. O., & Loftus, E. F. (2013). Are the "memory wars" over? A scientist-practitioner gap in beliefs about repressed memory. *Psychological Science, 25*(2), 519–530. https://doi.org/10.1177/0956797613510718

Rosenbaum, B., Jovic, V., & Varvin, S. (2020). Understanding the refugee-traumatised persons. *Psychosozial, 43*(3), 11–23.

Schreuder, B. J. N., van Egmond, M., Kleijn, W. C., & Visser, A. T. (1998). Daily reports of posttraumatic nightmares and anxiety dreams in Dutch war victims. *Journal of Anxiety Disorders, 12*(6), 511–524.

Shatan, C. F. (1972). *Post-Vietnam syndrome.* Retrieved February 8, 2018, from www.nytimes.com/1972/05/06/archives/postvietnam-syndrome.html

Shatan, C. F. (1973). The grief of soldiers: Vietnam combat veterans' self-help movement. *American Journal of Orthopsychiatry.* Shatan, Chaim F.: 415 Central Park West, New York, NY, US, 10025: American Orthopsychiatric Association, Inc.

Shephard, B. (2001). *The war on nerves: Soldiers and psychiatrists in the twentieth century.* Cambridge, MA: Harvard University Press.

Špirić, Ž. (2008). Psihoneurobiologija posttraumatskog stresnog poremećaja [Psychoneurobiology of posttraumatic stress disorder]. In Ž. Špirić (Ed.), *Ratna psihotrauma srpskih veterana* (pp. 181–200). Beograd: Udruženje boraca rata od 1990. godine i Čigoja štampa.

Špirić, Ž., Knežević, G., Jović, V., & Opačić, G. (2004). *Torture in war, consequences and rehabilitation of victims: Yugoslav experience.* Belgrade: IAN-International Aid Network.

Tindale, C. W. (1996). The logic of torture: A critical examination. *Social Theory and Practice, 22*(3), 349–374.

Varvin, S. (2017). Our relations to refugees: Between compassion and dehumanization. *The American Journal of Psychoanalysis, 77*(4), 359–377.

Weber, B. (2017). The EU-Turkey refugee deal and the not quite closed Balkan route. *Sarajevo.* Retrieved from http://library.fes.de/pdf-files/bueros/sarajevo/13436.pdf.

Young, A. (1995). *The harmony of illusions: Inventing post-traumatic stress disorder.* Princeton, NJ: Princeton University Press.

12 Long-term psychoanalytic treatments with traumatised refugees[1]

Sverre Varvin

Introduction

Refugees flee from war, persecution, torture, and other human rights violations (HRV); many meet extreme conditions during flight with maltreatment (also by police and border guards), rape, death, and extreme insecurity (Jovic, 2018), and many become severely traumatised. They are exposed to undefined waiting during flight and, as a rule, also when arriving in a country where they can seek asylum. Waiting is often experienced as a great mental pressure (Sagbakken et al., 2020). Western countries have now developed strategies of deterrence with strict border controls and policies aiming at keeping refugees away (EU, 2016; Gammeltoft-Hansen, 2016).

Research has shown an overrepresentation of mental health suffering among individuals with a refugee background compared to the majority population (Bogic et al., 2015; Fazel et al., 2005, 2012; Hassan et al., 2016; Hocking et al., 2015; Priebe et al., 2010; Sabes-Figuera et al., 2012), even after many years in a host country (Opaas et al., 2020; Vaage et al., 2010).

There is a high degree of resilience among refugees (Sleijpen et al., 2016; UNHCR, 2016), which is highly dependent on possibilities for treatment and making a decent life (Betancourt et al., 2015; Ungar, 2012; Varvin, 2015).

Children (approximately half of displaced persons), mothers with children, elders, and torture survivors are among the most vulnerable. Their basic needs and health care needs are often insufficiently covered, and traumatised refugees regularly wait for years before they get adequate treatment, if at all (Opaas & Varvin, 2015).

In this chapter I will describe the psychosocial situation of refugees and describe how psychoanalytic treatment may work for this often severely traumatised group of people.

Traumatisation

Traumatised persons struggle with mental and bodily pains difficult to understand and difficult to put into words. The pains may be expressed as dissociated states of mind, as bodily pains and other somatic experiences

DOI: 10.4324/9781003203223-14

and dysfunctions, as overwhelming thoughts and feelings, as behavioural tendencies and relational styles, as ways of living, and so forth. Traumatisation may be a causative and/or disposing factor in many psychopathological manifestations: depression, addiction, eating disorders, personality dysfunctions, and anxiety states (Leuzinger-Bohleber, 2012; Purnell, 2010; Taft et al., 2007; Vaage, 2010; Vitriol et al., 2009).

What is common are deficiencies in the representational system related to traumatic and other experiences; these experiences are painfully felt and set their marks on the body and the mind but are poorly contained in the mind. They are not or deficiently symbolised in the sense that they cannot be expressed in narratives in a way where meaning can emerge that can be reflected upon. They remain in the mind as dissociated or encapsulated fragments that have a disturbing effect on mood and mental stability (Rosenbaum & Varvin, 2007).

As a rule, extreme or complex traumatisation (like rape, torture) eludes meaning when it happens, and it precludes also forming an internal third position where the person, in his or her own mind, can create a reflecting distance to what is happening. The inner witnessing function, so vital for making meaning of experiences, is attacked during such extreme experiences, hindering the individual from being able to experience on a symbolic level the cruelties they have experienced.

Psychoanalytic treatment

How can people live through extreme and prolonged traumatisation, often in an extremely hostile environment, and how do they organise their lives in the aftermath? Understanding these processes give background to understand how derivatives related to the traumatising experiences manifest themselves in the therapeutic process. A main point is that the analyst, when taking on the task of treating such traumatised patients, inevitably becomes involved in the not-symbolised, fragmentary, and, as a rule, strongly affective scenarios related to the patient's traumatic experiences. This happens from the first encounter with the patient and is mostly expressed in the non-verbal interaction between the patient and the analyst. It may take a long time before these manifestations may be given a narrative form that in meaningful ways relates to traumatic and pretraumatic experiences, and it implies hard and painful emotional work from the patient, and from the analyst, to achieve this end.

Several therapeutic approaches (eg, EMDR, CBT) focus on PTSD, depression, and anxiety (Acarturk et al., 2015; Wong et al., 2015) so far with unconvincing results. I will here focus on psychoanalytic treatment, a treatment many severely traumatised persons prefer (van der Kolk et al., 1996). This user-based view on the advantages of psychoanalytic approaches was confirmed in research that demonstrated essential beneficiary aspects of psychodynamic therapy, as so-called evidence-based treatments had high dropout and non-responder rates (Schottenbauer et al., 2008a) and showed benefits from psychodynamic therapies for the following reasons (Schottenbauer et al., 2008b):

- They address crucial areas in the clinical presentation of PTSD and the sequels of trauma that are not targeted by current empirically supported treatments.
- They may be particularly helpful for complex PTSD, as they target problems related to the self and self-esteem, ability to resolve reactions to trauma through improved reflective functioning, and aim at the internalisation of more secure inner working models of relationships.
- They work on improving social functioning.
- They show continued improvement after treatment ends.

Patients with complex trauma often live in difficult social, economic, and cultural situations Treatment and rehabilitation, therefore, often need to be conducted by a team, and when and how to implement psychoanalytic therapy must be carefully evaluated and will need constant support from the team and other social services.

Trauma and the social context

For these not-symbolised and insufficiently symbolised experiences to approach some integration and be given some meaningful place in the individual's mind, they need to be actualised and given form in a holding and containing therapeutic relationship. This implies that the analyst must accept living with the patient in areas of the mind that are painfully absent of meaning and at times filled with horror. Further, without affirmation on the political, social, and cultural level, the traumatised person's feeling of unreality and fragmentation connected with the experiences may continue as has been the case for many groups: Holocaust survivors, war sailors, victims of genocides, and so on (Varvin, 2017).

The dynamic and structure of extreme traumatisation

How trauma affects a person depends on the severity; complexity and duration of the traumatising event; the context, whether intrafamilial or external; and the developmental stage. Central is the way in which traumatisation affects internal object relations – for example, whether earlier traumatic relations are activated and on the perceived support after the event and the treatment offered (Keilson & Sarpathie, 1979).

I will here concentrate on adult-onset trauma and give one example from a traumatised refugee in psychoanalytic therapy.

Phenomenology of traumatisation

Being traumatised is an experience of something unexpected that should not happen. It creates an internal situation of profound helplessness and an experience of being abandoned by all good and helping persons and internal objects. The feeling of helplessness and being abandoned may be carried over into the posttraumatic phase. A deep fear of an impending catastrophe of helplessness where nobody will help or care may develop. An inner feeling of desperation and fear of psychosomatic breakdown with fear of annihilation may ensue, and much of posttraumatic pathology may be seen as defence against and an attempt to cope with this impending catastrophe (Winnicott, 1991)

Human-made traumatisation influences internal object relation scenarios in different ways. Early traumas that bear similarity to the present traumatisation may be activated, making the present trauma imbued with earlier losses, humiliations, and traumatic experiences (Opaas & Varvin, 2015). Even early safe-enough relationships may be coloured by the later traumatising relationships when, for example, a too authoritarian father may be fused with a torturer, thus almost deleting the good-enough aspects of this relationship.

Complicated relations to the traumatising agent/person, the circumstances, and other relations involved may thus ensue, and these may be actualised in the transference.

The traumatised person internalises important aspects of the traumatising scenario in the form of self-object relation which may be more or often less differentiated and/or fragmented and in different ways self-negating. The actualisation of these may in the analytic process take dramatic forms.

Relation and symbolisation

One salient task in psychotherapy with traumatised patients is to enhance a metacognitive or mentalising capacity that can enable the patient to deal more effectively with traces and derivatives of the traumatic experience. This implies helping the patient out of mental states characterised by concreteness and lack of dimensionality.

During traumatisation the ego meets an overwhelming abundance of stimuli and impressions. The regulating functions of the mind breaks down, and the processes of the psychic apparatus are pushed towards states of extreme anxiety and catastrophe (Rosenbaum & Varvin, 2007). Mental traces of such traumatic experiences are "wild" in the sense that the person has no capacity to organise and deal with them, no inner container in a relation to an inner empathic other that can help give meaning to their experience (Laub, 2005).

There is an experience of loss of internal protection – primarily, the loss of the necessary feelings of basic trust and mastery. An empathic internal other is no longer functioning as a protective shield, and the functions that give meaning to experience may no longer work. Attachment to and trust in others may be perceived as dangerous reminding of previous catastrophes. Relating to others, for example, a psychoanalyst, may be felt as a risk of re-experiencing the original helplessness and a feeling of being left alone in utter despair. Withdrawal patterns may be the consequence, creating a negative spiral, as withdrawal at the same time means the loss of potential external support (Varvin & Rosenbaum, 2011).

Traumatisation may thus affect several dimensions of the person's relations with the external world and give disturbances on the bodily affective level, on the capacity to form relations with others and the group and family, and on the ability to give meaning to experience. The last is dependent on the social and cultural meaning-giving functions, which under normal circumstances provide affirmative narratives – for example, stories told by elders, scientific explanations (eg, psychological theories), and political acknowledgement (eg, leaders' acknowledging the historical circumstances of the atrocity).

The task of therapy is to allow these poorly mentalised experiences to emerge in the transference relationship so that words and meaning can be co-created even if the experiences themselves by all human standards are cruel and devoid of meaning.

The traumatising experiences must thus become actual in the therapeutic relationship. This may happen when the analyst is drawn into relational scenarios where he/she becomes part of the emerging trauma-related scenes that the patient hitherto has struggled with alone.

I will in the following pages demonstrate one aspect of psychoanalytic therapy that may be an important step in this symbolising process.

Actualisation, projective identification, and enactment

The traumatised patient will from the start of therapy involve the analyst in a not-symbolised and unconscious relationship where the patient communicates by acting out and in this way presents important aspects of their traumatic experiences (Varvin, 2013).

What the patient communicates touches the analyst and may hook on to the unconscious, not worked through the material on his/her side, resulting in action that, at first sight, is not therapeutic and is therefore named countertransference enactment (Jacobs, 1986).

Such enactments on the analyst's side may, however, be a starting point for a possible process of symbolisation and becoming conscious of these implicit experiences (Scarfone, 2011).

An enactment involves a collapse in the therapeutic dialogue where the analyst is drawn into an interaction where she or he unwittingly acts, thereby actualising unconscious wishes of both himself or herself and the patient. It may be a definable episode in a process with more or less clear distinctions between the pre-phase, the actual moment, and the post-phase but may also be part of a prolonged process in therapy (Jacobs, 1986). Enactment appears thus as an unintentional breakdown of the analytic rule of "speech not act," and this may imply a new opportunity of integration, or it may hinder the analytic process when it goes unnoticed or unanalysed.

Enactments may represent a possibility for symbolising material related to traumatic experiences and lay the ground for remembering, not only "recalling" or "evoking." It implies the transmutation of some material into a new form in order to be brought into the psychic field where the functions of remembering and integration can occur (Scarfone, 2011).

Enactments can thus in this context be seen as actualisation of relational scripts or scenarios where unconscious, not-symbolised material are activated both in the patient and in the analyst. This is seen as an unavoidable part of the analytic interaction, and the outcome depends on the analytic couple's ability to bring the enactment into the psychic field.

I will briefly illustrate aspects of these processes.

Loss and trauma – a case story

F, a woman in her late thirties, came to Norway as a refugee from a country in the Middle East nine years prior to treatment. She was in psychoanalytic psychotherapy face to face, two to three times a week, for one and a half years.

She reported a relatively happy childhood. She was married and was working as clerk when she was arrested for participating in a non-violent political organisation together with her husband. At the time of her arrest, she was pregnant in the last trimester. She was maltreated physically (including beatings on her pregnant womb, threats, seclusion, etc.) and suffered from malnutrition and lack of proper medical care when she became ill. Her husband was arrested at the same time and was tortured to death some months later. She was allowed to go to a public hospital to give birth, and an escape was arranged for her shortly thereafter. While she was living clandestinely, her child died of an unknown disease, probably caused by the torture, maltreatment, and lack of adequate medical care during her stay in prison.

After the death of her child and husband, she lived clandestinely for about one year before she fled from her country under difficult circumstances. During this time, she experienced additional serious traumas.

She arrived in Norway severely depressed and suicidal and had serious eating problems in addition to posttraumatic symptoms and psychosomatic symptoms. In the years in Norway, she suffered almost continuously from nightmares, re-experiencing, avoidance behaviour, somatisation, and psychosomatic illness and recurrent depressions. Despite this, she managed to settle and achieve a considerable degree of integration in the community. She lived alone and had friends but no intimate contact with men. High levels of activity, lots of helping others, and little time for herself, seemingly reflecting a need to act rather than feel, characterised her life in exile.

F had to a large extent mourned her husband, for example, performing grief-rituals on his birthday. The loss of her child was not a problem she presented when seeking therapy, and it remained silent during the first part until it emerged in a quite dramatic way in a session after a week's break in the treatment.

She arrived on time at the session, out of breath, as she had been running believing she was late. Her first remark was, "I lost the bus" (A common expression in Norwegian when coming late for the bus, and here also indicating the theme of loss). In the first part of the session, she spoke in a staccato manner evoking a strong need in the analyst to help and support her.

She talked about her loneliness during the break, the need to have someone to lean on, to trust, and who could be close. The analyst affirmed her feeling of loneliness and her longing for a family. She then defended against this by idealising a more independent life. Her own family and her close relations to them and also her ambivalent feelings towards them had been a theme throughout the therapy. In this section of the session, the analyst's interventions also became intellectual with lack of affective resonance. The analyst did in this way join the patient in an enactment attempting to ward off painful material.

Then a shift occurred when the analyst remarked, remembering her earlier clearly stated affection for her family, that they, her family, surely would have liked her to establish a family in exile. She then became silent for some minutes and said crying:

"Yes, I have been thinking if I had my son, he would have been 10 years old and . . . "

She cried much and seemed distant, obviously re-experiencing scenes from the past. She then haltingly, in short sentences, and after encouragement, talked about the birth of her child, how happy she had been when she heard the child cry. It was felt like a victory. Also, the dangers came to her mind, and she was frightened and desperate in the session. She did not manage to stop crying as she left.

This was a breakthrough of memories, or rather a "recalling" or "evoking," which came as a surprise for the patient (and for the analyst). It was a re-experiencing "like a film" of the traumatic scenario, a broken narrative.

She was physically ill during the night, and when she came the next day, she was still quite affected, and it gradually became clear what had happened before and during the previous sessions, which in fact represented an actualisation of the drama when she lost her child.

Three consecutive nights before the key session she had had the following dream, which she told, realising the connection with her child's death:

And then suddenly I get all; I feel I, I got like; I had/I did not tell you,
    I dreamt for three nights [before the key session] that I cried. . . .
I was very narrow in my throat and, and had like saliva around my mouth. It's like a; then I thought like, what is it that makes me feel. I don't get enough oxygen and (heavy breathing), when I, eh, was in the middle of crying, when I woke up.
    She then could narrate how her child died:

She was living clandestinely in poor conditions. Her child got fever and had increasing difficulties in breathing. In the end the baby died in her arms of lack of air (asphyxia). Her despair and grief were abruptly interrupted by the dangerous circumstances, which demanded that she move on. Her baby was buried in haste, and the harsh tone among her comrades stopped any attempt from her for emotional reactions.

We can now reconstruct aspects of what happened in her therapy.[2] She had a markedly positive, almost idealising transference towards the analyst. In the break she had felt utmost lonely, and this had evoked in her unconscious memories of her child as well as other persons she had lost (her husband and also her father, who died when she was in exile). In the session she came out of breath with a feeling of loss (expressed in her first remark: "I lost the bus"). The countertransference was characterised by a desperate wish to help but then a felt helplessness, which resulted in distancing and intellectualisation on the analyst's side.

In hindsight it was possible to identify several episodes earlier in the therapy where the theme of loss had come up and also where dead children had been mentioned. This had obviously been small attempts by the patient to bring maybe her most painful experience into the therapy, but she then backed away and either intellectualised or dropped the theme. The analyst had colluded with this and avoided the theme of loss, which had connection with the analyst's own problems and some unresolved issues concerning his own losses. These countertransference problems were possible to identify, understand, and reflect on only when analysing the sessions afterwards.

The theme of loss became, however, more acute for her in the break preceding this key session. She had obviously during this time, partly unconsciously, lived through and been occupied with her tragic loss and identified with her dead child and, by projective identification, the analyst got the role of the helpless helper, pushing him to act according to the role assigned to this part. This interpretation was supported by analyst's subjective countertransference reactions (ie, feeling solicitous but helpless).

The relative abstinence in the session allowed her to start symbolising her traumatic loss. The dreams were obviously a signal of an unconscious preparation for re-experiencing the death of her child, in which she gave voice to the part of herself identified with the child trying to survive.

As the loss theme was elaborated, F began to integrate the loss of her child with her other losses – her husband's death, her father's death some years ago, and also other deaths. Thus, the emergence of the loss of her child brought with it memories of other losses, which she then worked to integrate and mourn during the rest of the therapy. She also had to face her guilt for not having been able to help her child, which may be interpreted as survivor's guilt.

Needless to say, this was a hard and laborious process also for the analyst who had to work on his own unresolved issues. The work was not completed, but the treatment did make a difference in her life; she was no longer depressed and had less somatic pain and, more importantly, she started a new way of life. She was no longer the tireless helper; she took time to care for herself and relax, and she managed to establish a relationship with a man.

Discussion

F's experiences in her therapeutic process reflect complex interactions on a verbal and non-verbal level. Traumatic experiences are present in the mind and body of the traumatised in different ways, all seeking expression in communicative styles and ways of being in relation to the analyst. They may dramatically involve the analyst in processes that touch the analyst's own unresolved or partly resolved issues and draw him into a process of acting instead of thinking and reflecting. The transference-countertransference situation may push the analyst to become involved in a relational scenario that, as a rule, is possible to understand and interpret only after the fact. In the sequence presented from F's treatment, the analyst became the "helpless helper" in the transference and defended against this feeling by joining the patient's intellectualisation. The transference situations vary, and different personas from the patient's internal world may appear in the transference as, for example, the perpetrator, the dehumanised victim, and so forth.

It is argued that countertransference enactment may be a central vehicle for unsymbolised trauma-related material to emerge and that when this happens, an opportunity may appear for the "unthought known" to be heard and contained in a joint created narrative that relates present suffering to past misery. A time-dimension can then be established in this area of the psyche, which also makes reflection possible. The precondition is attention to countertransference reactions and fantasies and the analyst's capacity for containment and gradual reflection and working though of the personal part of his reactions.

What happens is a mostly unconscious "mis en scene," which may happen over a longer time in therapy. What we saw in this example was a more acute reaction of the analyst, but also that avoiding the loss theme probably had been going on for a prolonged part of the treatment.

Traumatised persons' experiences represent a partial foreclosure where parts of the symbolic function are undermined. Foreclosed signifiers are not integrated in the subject's unconscious, so they tend to re-emerge from the outside, in "the Real" (Lacan, 1977). Another way of saying this is that they appear as beta elements and sometimes also as bizarre object experiences as coming from the outside through, for example, hallucinations (Bion, 1977). These mechanisms may also be reflected in traumatised persons' attention and concentration problems and their difficulties in organising impressions in thoughts (van der Kolk, 2014). Many traumatised persons have, moreover, experienced that language was perverted during torture and other atrocity situations, which have the consequence that they, to a large degree, have learned to rely on non-verbal communication. In torture, for example, everyday expressions are often used for the most gruesome torture practices; confusing communications are used to break down people.

The fact that so much of the focus in interpersonal relations with severely traumatised patients rely on the non-verbal dimensions may explain to a certain extent why many traumatised patients feel safe in a "psychoanalytic context" and why psychoanalytic therapy works when patient and analyst have different cultural backgrounds and different native languages.

Massive traumatisation creates destabilisation of the basic structures of human relationships:

- On the level of intimate relationships where intrapsychic and interpersonal functions concern regulations of emotions, primary care functions, and basic identity issues.
- On the level of the individual relations to the group where personal identity and developmental tasks are negotiated.
- On the cultural or discourse level, where narratives are established that give meaning to and stabilise relations and developments on the individual and group levels (Rosenbaum & Varvin, 2007).

Any approach to patients who have been traumatised in a violent social context, such as wars, mass persecution, and genocides, must therefore be sensitive to and take into consideration the dimensions of social and cultural influences on development, psychopathology, and health-sickness behaviour.

Lack of social support and recognition has for many traumatised persons been devastating. Treatment of traumatised patients can therefore only with great difficulty work in a social/cultural setting where traumatisation is not acknowledged and worked with at other levels in society.

Notes

1 This chapter is based on material from my book: *Psychoanalysis in Social and Cultural Settings. Upheavals and Resilience* (Varvin, 2021).
2 The therapy process was analysed longitudinally using assimilation analysis. This analysis tracks the development of problematic experiences throughout therapy through a qualitative procedure using narrative and procedural aspects of the therapeutic dialogue (Varvin, 2003; Varvin & Stiles, 1999).

References

Acarturk, C., Konuk, E., Cetinkaya, M., Senay, I., Sijbrandij, M., Cuijpers, P., & Aker, T. (2015). EMDR for Syrian refugees with posttraumatic stress disorder symptoms: Results of a pilot randomized controlled trial. *European Journal of Psychotraumatology, 6.* doi:10.3402/ejpt.v6.27414.

Betancourt, T. S., Abdi, S., Ito, B. S., Lilienthal, G. M., Agalab, N., & Ellis, H. (2015). We left one war and came to another: Resource loss, acculturative stress, and caregiver-child relationships in Somali refugee families. *Cultural Diversity & Ethnic Minority Psychology, 21*(1), 114–125. http://dx.doi.org/10.1037/a0037538.

Bion, W. (1977). *Seven servants*. New York: Aronson.

Bogic, M., Njoku, A., & Priebe, S. (2015). Long-term mental health of war-refugees: a systematic literature review. *BMC International Health and Human Rights*, 15–29. doi:10.1186/s12914-015-0064-9

EU. (2016). *European commission – Fact sheet*. Retrieved from http://europa.eu/rapid/press-release_MEMO-16-963_en.htm.

Fazel, M., Reed, R., Panter-Brick, C., & Stein, A. (2012). Mental health of displaced and refugee children resettled in high-income countries: Risk and protective factors. *The Lancet, 379,* 266–282. doi:10.1016/S0140-6736(11)60051-2

Fazel, M., Wheeler, J., & Danesh, J. (2005). Prevalence of serious mental disorder in 7000 refugees resettled in western countries: A systematic review. *The Lancet, 365,* 1309–1314.

Gammeltoft-Hansen, T. (2016). *Hvordan løser vi flyktningkrisen?* København: Information forlag.

Hassan, G., Ventevogel, P., Jefee-Bahloul, H., Barkil-Oteo, A., & Kirmayer, L. J. (2016). Mental health and psychosocial wellbeing of Syrians affected by armed conflict. *Epidemiology and Psychiatric Sciences, 25*(2), 129–141.

Hocking, D. C., Kennedy, G. A., & Sundram, S. (2015). Mental disorders in asylum seekers: The role of the refugee determination process and employment. *Journal of Nervous and Mental Disease, 203*(1), 28–32. doi:http://dx.doi.org/10.1097/NMD.0000000000000230

Jacobs, T. (1986). On countertransference enactments. *Journal of the American Psychoanalytic Association, 34,* 289–307.

Jovic, V. (2018). Working with traumatized refugees on the Balkan route. *International Journal of Applied Psychoanalytic Studies, 15*(3), 187–201. doi:10.1002/aps.1586.

Keilson, H., & Sarpathie, R. (1979). *Sequentieller Traumatisierung bei Kindern*. Stuttgart: Ferdinand Enke.

Lacan, J. (1977). *Écrits*. Hammondsworth: Penguin Books.

Laub, D. (2005). Traumatic shutdown of narrative and symbolization: A death instinct derivative? *Contemporary Psychoanalysis, 41*(2), 307–326.

Leuzinger-Bohleber, M. (2012). Changes in dreams – From a psychoanalysis with a traumatised, chronic depressed patient. In H. K. Peter Fonagy, M. Leuzinger-Bohleber, & D. Taylor (Eds.), *The significance of dreams* (pp. 49–88). London: Karnac Books.

Opaas, M., & Varvin, S. (2015). Relationships of childhood adverse experiences with mental health and quality of life at treatment start for adult refugees traumatized by pre-flight experiences of war and human rights violations. *Journal of Nervous and Mental Disease, 203*(9), 684–695. http://dx.doi.org/10.1097/NMD.0000000000000330

Opaas, M., Wentsel Larsen, T., & Varvin, S. (2020). The 10-year course of mental health, quality of life, and exile life functioning in traumatized refugees from treatment start. *PLoS One, 15*(2). doi:e0244730. https://doi.org/10.1371/journal.pone.0244730

Priebe, S., Bogic, M., Ashcroft, R., Franciskovic, T., Galeazzi, G., Kucukalic, A., . . . Ajdukovic, D. (2010). Experience of human rights violations and subsequent mental disorders – A study following the war in the Balkans. *Social Science & Medicine, 71*, 2170–2177.

Purnell, C. (2010). Childhood trauma and adult attachment. *Healthcare Counselling and Psychotherapy Journal, 20*(2).

Rosenbaum, B., & Varvin, S. (2007). The influence of extreme traumatisation on body, mind and social relations. *International Journal of Psychoanalysis, 88*, 1527–1542.

Sabes-Figuera, R., McCrone, P., Bogic, M., Ajdukovic, D., Franciskovic, T., Colombini, N., . . . Priebe, S. (2012, January). Long-term impact of war on healthcare costs: An eight-country study. *PLoS One, 7*(1), ArtID e29603. http://dx.doi.org/10.1371/journal.pone.0029603

Sagbakken, M., Bregård, I., & Varvin, S. (2020). The past, the present, and the future: A qualitative study exploring how refugees' experience of time influences their mental health and well-being. *Frontiers in Sociology*. doi:10.3389/fsoc.2020.00046.

Scarfone, D. (2011). Repetition: Between presence and meaning. *Canadian Journal of Psychoanalysis/Revue canadienne de psychoanalyse, 19*(1), 70–86.

Schottenbauer, M., Glass, C., Arnkoff, D., & Gray, S. (2008a). Contributions of psychodynamic approaches to treatment of PTSD and trauma: A review of the empirical treatment and psychopathology literature. *Psychiatry, 71*(1), 13–34.

Schottenbauer, M., Glass, C., Arnkoff, D., Tendick, V., & Gray, S. (2008b). Nonresponse and dropout rates in outcome studies on PTSD: Review and methodological considerations. *Psychiatry, 71*(2), 134–168.

Sleijpen, M., Boeije, H. R., Kleber, R. J., & Mooren, T. (2016). Between power and powerlessness: A meta-ethnography of sources of resilience in young refugees. *Ethn Health, 21*(2), 158–180.

Taft, C., Kaloupek, D., Schumm, J., Marshall, A., Panuzio, J., King, D., & Keane, T. (2007). Posttraumatic stress disorder symptoms, physiological reactivity, alcohol problems, and aggression among military veterans. *Journal of Abnormal Psychology, 116*(3), 498–507.

Ungar, M. E. (2012). *The social ecology of resilience. A handbook of theory and practice.* New York, Dordrecht, Heidelberg, and London: Springer Verlag.

UNHCR. (2016). *Regional refugee & resilience plan 2016–2017. In response to the Syria crisis.* Retrieved from www.unhcr.org/54918efa9.html.

Vaage, A. B. (2010). Long-term mental health of Vietnamese refugees in the aftermath of trauma. *The British Journal of Psychiatry, 196,* 122–125.

Vaage, A. B., Thomsen, P. H., Silove, D., Wentzel-Larsen, T., Van Ta, T., & Hauff, E. (2010). Long-term mental health of Vietnamese refugees in the aftermath of trauma. *British Journal of Psychiatry, 196,* 122–125.

van der Kolk, B. A. (2014). *The body keeps the score. Mind, brain and body in transformation of trauma.* London: Allen Lane, and imprint of Penguin Books.

van der Kolk, B. A., McFarlane, A. C., & Weisaeth, L. (1996). *Traumatic stress.* New York and London: The Guilford Press.

Varvin, S. (2003). *Mental survival strategies after extreme traumatisation.* Copenhagen: Multivers.

Varvin, S. (2013). Trauma als nonverbaler kommunikation. *Zeitschrift für psychoanalytische Theorie und Praxis, 28,* 114–130.

Varvin, S. (2015). Trauma and resilience. In G. Leo (Ed.), *Psychoanalysis, collective traumas and memory places.* Lecce, Italy: Frenis Zero.

Varvin, S. (2017). Our relations to refugees: Between compassion and dehumanization. *The American Journal of Psychoanalysis, 77*(4), 1–19.

Varvin, S. (2021). *Psychoanalysis in social and cultural settings. Upheavals and resilience.* New York: Routledge.

Varvin, S., & Rosenbaum, B. (2011). Severely traumatized patients' attempts at reorganizing their relations to others in psychotherapy: An enunciation analysis In N. Freedman, M. Hurvich, & R. Ward (Eds.), *Another kind of evidence. Studies on internalization, annihilation anxiety, and progressive symbolization in the psychoanalytic process* (pp. 226–243). London: Karnac Books.

Varvin, S., & Stiles, W. B. (1999). Emergence of severe traumatic experiences: An assimilation analysis of a psychoanalytic therapy with a political refugee. *Psychotherapy Research, 9*(3), 381–404. Retrieved from www.tandf.co.uk/journals/titles/10503307.asp

Vitriol, V. B., Florenzano, R. U., Weil, K. P., & Benadof, D. F. (2009). Evaluation of an outpatient intervention for women with severe depression and a history of childhood trauma. *Psychiatric Services, 60,* 936–942.

Winnicott, D. W. (1991). [Fear of breakdown]. *Psyche, 45*(12), 1116–1126. Retrieved from PM:1775645

Wong, E. C., Marshall, G. N., Schell, T. L., Berthold, S., & Hambarsoomians, K. (2015). Characterizing the mental health care of U.S. Cambodian refugees. *Psychiatric Services, 66*(9), 980–984. http://dx.doi.org/10.1176/appi.ps.201400368

13 Fifteen years of psychoanalytical fieldwork in Eastern African cities

Barbara Saegesser

Introduction

In all these Eastern African cities – Alexandria, Khartoum, Addis Ababa, Djibouti, Uganda, Stone Town – from Egypt to the Indian Ocean, where I worked in places and institutions such as very different orphanages, drop-ins for street boys, hospitals for the poorest ones, maternity (with genitally mutilated women in the third degree), central hospitals and psychiatric departments, I stayed in situations where the enormous need prevailed. I selected the particular area for my work myself; for example, in the maternal care unit, I have chosen to work with pregnant women in labour, the ones going through critical childbirths (because of genital mutilation in the third degree), in the preparation room, in the operation theatre, post-op recovery, or the neonatal unit.

Currently, I was in the main hospital and psychiatry department. As soon as I arrive, they tell me that it is up to me to choose with which of the "difficult patients" I wish to work. I am immediately directed to the "difficult patients" and asked to "do something with them." These patients are children – orphans accompanied by aunt or grandmother – and women, men, people with drug addictions, or suffering from malnutrition and, of course, the daily misery of people who are psychosomatically affected.

In comparison to patients in European clinics, the individual conditions of the East African patients in psychiatric and other fields of medical help and environment are not comparable. I work in Eastern Africa in much more miserable and dramatic situations. With the young doctors in all these hospitals, I try to form a Balint group and accompany them, whenever possible, during their rounds to see the patients and discuss about diagnostics. During my diverse orphanage and hospital work with children, adults, and even some of their caregivers who are suffering from extreme psychosomatic distress, I have become familiar with many cultural and cultural-religious characteristics about East African political-religious and ethnic groups. Furthermore, I have gained much experience with young orphans, older war orphans, people threatened by hunger and fear, and those gravely marked by psychosomatic suffering – especially,

DOI: 10.4324/9781003203223-15

intern African refugees in Eastern Africa. The latter are mainly from Somalia, Sudan, Eritrea, and Ethiopia. At the same time, I learned to treasure in a new way my psychoanalytic concepts and clinical experience that also built the essential basis for my work in Eastern Africa. I am confronted by the most alarming forms of psychic and psychosomatic illnesses and disease and near-death conditions.

Psychoanalytic interpretation of experiences

After some time of working in my field, I have started to realise that in many places, psychology is hardly known and not at all practiced, and natural psychotherapy even less. I am getting used to the fact that with my psychoanalytic approach, thinking and evaluating configurations, I am bringing something foreign to a particular culture or ethnic group and also to an individual's comprehension and self-understanding or to a family structure. This means that I not only have to face the distrust against white people who want to "apply" something unfamiliar, that can remind one heavily of colonial actions. At the same time, I am confronted with mistrust caused by the way I approach and interact with babies, children, and adults – primarily women – and work with them psychoanalytically. The terms "psychotherapy" and the "psychosomatic" themselves are unknown, even in the medical and psychiatric care fields.

In general, my experience in the parts of East Africa where I have been active is that despite the cultural differences and difficulties, it is nevertheless possible to work in all these places. I apply my knowledge about very difficult and sensible issues, and I'm weighing carefully which of my thoughts to share and which not. Working this way, patients are beginning to become interested in themselves and others, perhaps even in a new way. Something begins to shift.

The individual, subjective psyche is predominantly ignored in many Eastern African political-religious, cultures, and ethnic groups. Politics and Islamic religion go from the beginning of this religion together. There is no secular separation of both. The "own" psychic process is formed accordingly to the Koran, as its teachings should – and apparently can – regulate and fulfil all individual human subjective and "objective" needs, including psychic ones.

I do not represent any ideology, at least not outwardly. By my approach with its intensive, therapeutic mirroring function, my "reverie" of my patients and my personal hypotheses about them and their psychic configuration, I can try to provide them somehow "a little freedom" in their thinking, that allows them to discover something very tiny, that is new – that is, found again – that can develop and grow. This might be, for example, the ability to discriminate or perceive something either "new or already known" in a way that allows patients to unfold apparently as "unfamiliar," in some way dangerous seen desires and wishes.

These new aspects of the non-Islamic formed world of thinking and feeling, especially the unconscious, rediscovered psychic qualities do not accord with the norms and rituals in and of the Koran, regarding the thinking and feeling of people who are Muslim.

Those issues are thought to work in a more or less psychoanalytical way with refugees and migrants who have suffered and gone through other countries – they fortunately did not die – during their fight to survive and during their flight.

It seems important to me *not* to think that a refuge should be grateful to be in a safe land, where the chances to develop his or her own life in a much better way, than before the horror of his or her flight, are per se given. He or she often is not grateful but deeply disappointed, because he or she expected and did hope during all the horrible flight away from his or her homeland to arrive finally more or less in paradise.

The *religious* background should in every case be known. For refugees from Eastern Africa this is much more important, as, for example, for refugees from Western Africa. Some knowledge of the specific religious and cultural background is absolutely vital.

Refugees from Eastern Africa seemed to be *more closely* attached to religions like the Koran/Islam (and some natural religions) than refugees from Western Africa. One of the reasons for this religious attachment may be their fundamental precarious circumstances in their daily life. They live near the Sahel. In many African countries religion and politics are always interconnected. There exist Islamic laws and rules that are valid for everybody, and their position goes over the "normal" juristic laws (ie, the Koranic Lex of Sharia; Sunna; and the five columns of Islam: Schahāda, Salāt, Zakat, Saum, Haddsch.) Neglecting Koranic laws can mean being killed or enduring lifelong negative consequences, especially for women. They can be killed by stoning or excluded from the familiar and the whole society, thus suffering by their social death.

The psychotherapist's gender is very important for the patient she or he is working with. For a Muslim man it is most difficult to hear and accept the word of women. For a Muslim woman it is usual and goes with the line of her life, designed by her God, to hear and accept the word of a man.

A *man* has the first position in the system of the world; women have the second position. A man is, as a man, nearer to God. A husband orders what his wife has to do and be. Concerning sexual attitudes, a man can take, if he wishes to do so, a woman for what is in his mind, for what he likes to do. Respect towards a *woman* is not really demanded, especially if the woman is not married. A woman on the other hand should show and behave herself as a not-sexual, asexual person, as a person not having sexual wishes. And besides all this, the *"umma,"* the whole family structure, that goes over some 1,000 km – for example from the Indian Ocean to the northeast of Ethiopia – is fundamentally important.

The narcissistic and gender value of women is very small or somewhat like nothing, besides other manipulation, for example, by genital mutilation of women in the third degree (named Pharaonic), especially in Somalia. That means the clitoris is cut away, the inner and outer labias are cut away, and the vaginal opening is sewn together except for a small opening, as small as a hazelnut, just for leak menstrual blood and urine and to take in male seeds. This third degree of mutilation is mainly performed in Somalia. This and other forms of genital mutilation find practice in Eastern Africa. Women have got the ability and the "religious order" to hide difficulties – for example, genital mutilation. It seems to be clear that their deep feelings of shame are involved in their somewhat mute and masochistic ways of communication.

The topic of "time" is fundamentally different. Time is always there, as it would be and given in an infinite way. Time is never short or too short; it is given and has no end. Time can – symbolically seen – in Eastern Africa never be money, just as in other parts of the world. Money is in East African regions not "given." Money is connected with the model of "always too little." This fact influences the inner relation to work for money, to be a working man/working woman and to daily work for earning one's living.

Body and soul questions and problems of a human being are in the hands of God. There is no model of an individual human being as we see it in Western societies or also in our psychoanalytical concepts of a psychosomatic individual. The Islamic and psychoanalytic worlds are by trend two different worlds. We should not forget this when working with Muslim refugees. Muslim patients often do not see and feel themselves as a subject who can wish and act more or less fully himself or herself. God is making him or her go this or another or a third way. The centre of the life of a Muslim is his god, Allah, or the prophet Mohammed. Allah is thinking for and conducting men and women. A human being has, corresponding to the holy Islamic writings, not got explicitly a psyche, a "psychisme."

I refer to refugees from Alexandria (Egypt), Khartoum (Sudan), Addis Ababa and Hawassa (Ethiopia), Djibouti, Kampala (Uganda), Stone Town (Tanzania). All these refugees have nearly the same background as refugees from Eritrea (in this case with politically fascist totalitarian impact from the regime, which can trigger specific anxiety and paranoid) – in European terms and meaning – reactions and Somalia (the intense anxiety reactions due primarily because of the deadly actions of Al-Shabaab), and the same anxiety and somehow paranoid reactions can characterise refugees from South Sudan and DRCongo (in both countries, women are dramatically suffering or dying by gender – that is, from genital-based rape) and also the Central African Republic.

Refugees who had to spend a long time in their flight – two to three years – have mostly changed some characteristics of their personality on this long and harmful way to the paradisiacal country they think to come. If they are able, they can learn much in their flight because they are together with people who are also fleeing from their own country from many parts of the world. They learn languages, customs, ways of thinking and life, and also to say or do what they think could be opportune to them. And when they finally arrive in the country they did dream of, the paradise-like one, they are overwhelmed by a terrible big deception. It is not so much grief as psychoanalysts might think, but, for instance, the terrible reality that they cannot help their family back home by sending money or pay back the money with which they found to help them to flee to a "good and rich country."

Refugees from Western African areas are in cultural, ethnic, and religious-political ways quite different. Several Western African countries are, by tendency, more open and interested in "Western matters" (including American thinking, showing, behaviour) than Eastern African societies, as far as I have seen. Eastern African societies, from Egypt down to the Indian Ocean, tend to be more conventional since a terrible deep poverty is definitely more common (the Zone of Sahel is nearby). And poverty can and does attach people to their religious structures and promises. Those promise hope of a better life on earth or after life on earth, in heaven. Some words and suras of the Koran are taken very literally, even if the result may be for European or American eyes very cruel (see the killing and mutilation of girls/women).

In many aspects, a refugee has seen and suffered much more than most of "us" European or American "Psy's," who have not suffered from flight and deadly threat. Often the *colour of a refugee's* body is not the same *as* "ours," and the language can be very, very different to the point of at first not understanding each other. This completely new situation may effect more or less consciously – on both sides of the therapeutic couple – deep feelings of anxiety, impotence, and despair. And consequently, one could try to ignore and trivialise this inconvenient and adverse inner status by thinking he comes from the dark/white continent; he's a little bit "unheimlich" – scary to me. He is worth less than me. Perhaps one then thinks well, he or she is to be pitied. To think this way, moreover, is not very fruitful for psychoanalytical work. In this modus we are not at the same level, and it would be important to do psychoanalytical work together. We lose the egalitarian optic of the patient. It is not an optimal start of psychoanalytical "team" work.

As a non-Eastern African man/woman and psychoanalyst, it is not favourable to think and feel as if you know more than the refugee or migrant. He or she knows himself surely better than you do and what you think you know about him or her.

One does not know more because of knowing about new technologies and so on. And I think it is not adequate to explain to her/him "what the world is and means." Our sight of the things of the world and experiences are very "other". To an African woman or man, it doesn't mean anything positive; sometimes it causes deep anxiety to stay alone in one room. Migrants from Eastern Africa are used to and like being surrounded by family and others just as they are most of the time also during their flight. To see planted flowers in a garden does not mean the same for migrants as for US or European people. Contrarily, it can be an object of deep envy: the white people have even money for those strange flowers. Don't think that what's a pleasure or dreadful for "us" means the same for migrants. His or her anxiety and pleasure registers are different. One of those intense pleasures seems to be his or her religious Islamic devotion – that is, five prayers a day and to leave everything about his or her life in the hands of the god Allah.

It is very possible that the knowledge the refugee has or had (before his traumatism due to his/her flight) contains other registers than the knowing about him or her of the psychoanalyst. I think of registers that are fully unknown and uncommon by a Christian-thinking psychoanalyst and that have to do with the Islamic political religion, magic thinking (natural religions), with completely other ethnic structures, also with inner structures, due to the orientations and fixation by Koranic suras and laws. It makes sense not to try to measure or see structures from the refugee through "Western" eyes and models of psyche. We should be able to follow all the movements – inner and outer – the migrant does show us, also in some sort of inner imitation movements by us. It is important to try to accept and to be interested in the registers the refugee shows us, I mean the ones that we do not know at all. The Islamic religion gives the refugee much inner holding. It can happen that he says to us, full of hope to be accepted this way by us, that he is not relying on his religion any more. Refugees are more or less forced to say what they think "we" (US and Western people) would like to hear, just to find themselves in a more comfortable position. It could be a way for them to see and arrange that they are not sent back home to their country.

It seems to be very important to give much time in the psychotherapeutic process to the refugee and to ourselves. It is important to be able to sustain this completely new situation; it is a stranger situation than we mostly face in our daily practice. And it is very important to see and let it be this way, if ever a refugee says his god, Allah, will look after him. This is what he really thinks in his very inner "soul," and this gives him inner holding, even if this is not what we think or see as an inner holding by a good evaluated self. Our theory of a "self" is fully at the other side or even averse to the Islamic religious-political inner feelings. Allah is absolutely the first "Figure" and has got the very first position in a man's or a woman's life. If we do think and believe in a very other way, we do not have the right to minimise the worth of Islamic thinking. In a therapeutic process, I think, we have to accept the "other" and understand that the patient as an individual has beliefs that are of as much value to him/her as ours are to us. This is not easy. I hear sometimes colleagues saying: "oh, that's not difficult, I do not need to know anything about Islam and those practices. Patients do follow without any problems my thinking." Well, they mostly do because they wish to be "a good patient." And some colleagues do not realise this; I mean that we can help to build another *faux self*.

If it is not possible to exchange verbally, the possibility exists to exchange without words or also with drawings. Do not use a translator right away. Last thing to remember, as is well known, they often mix their own thinking and ethnic problems in the translation. Sometimes they think to understand and communicate in a more sensitive and meaningful way than we do. Somehow this idea might be correct, but it does not play together with the psychotherapeutic exchange. And on the other hand, it is always possible a refugee does not trust another man or woman or a neighbour of his home country, especially if the person is an official-in-charge in the new country, where the exchange does happen.

By non-verbal exchange, all postures, all signs of a refugee – eyes, ears, lips, structure and form of the body, smell and vapour (and perhaps some very few words, if you understand their language) – are most important to see and to give. The most important moment in those therapies – just as in every one – is to hear and understand what the migrant does tell us, in any language ever. And that we stay in our psychoanalytic mode and inner setting.

In this special, non-verbal exchange, an ancient form of exchange that has to do with the beginning of our lives, every movement of the body, especially also vivid movement of the hands and, as I said, eyes, mouth, nose, and so on play an important role in making a beginning of "knowing" and vice versa. One can learn to come to a greater understanding of the inner traumatism of what suffering are affecting the refugee, when we are open enough to hear our unconscious. And in a second time we can perhaps introduce more formal psychoanalytical structures by performing it step by step. Sometimes we do not stay in our own space (room) of practice. Fortunately, we have got our own psychoanalytical setting in ourselves.

What we should absolutely avoid is to not to make *any acting out*, no sexual or other encroachments. Although those encounters may initially not be very fruitful, even hard to take, one should not react with too much reluctance, power, or sadism. Often, this reaction happens at times when we are going to be excessively frustrated and feel deeply helpless and impotent. In those moments we may fall into – or our unconscious may select – such a form of exchange. One can see it in the terrible near-death and sadistic forms of exchanges in refugee camps. They should be shelters for refugees all over the world, but the "helpers" are sometimes unable to act appropriately, because of unconscious wishes.

One form of this destructive acting is mostly gender specific and happens to women – seldom to men – as refugees or in flight: they are raped by one or several men. Rapists do this also with dangerous objects, with guns, bottlenecks and broken bottlenecks, and pieces of trees or other methods. All this may be done before the eyes of their children. It seems to be a perverse attempt to distance the lost or refugee women by harming her, destroying her, by making her as "worth nothing," not human and feeling deeply ashamed. Sometimes in a session with refugees, as a form of projective transfer, a therapist could see this very stranger in front of him as "unheimlich," scary and uncanny, as no longer a human being. In those moments sadism and negative power may enter into the treatment.

I write about all these terrible sexual brutal actions with the hope that we can avoid them. And because many female refugees, especially from South Sudan and the region of Kivu (DRC) could survive such brutal and near-to-death actions. They do hope for a new, much better way of life. All the refugees, especially women, often have been brutally raped already in their home countries and several times during their flight that created big traumatic narcissistic flaws, by especially genital mutilation. And it might be they think – more or less unconsciously – that sex is always demanded from them to make situations better and try to manoeuvre the psychoanalytical process in an erotic direction.

The obligation and inner surety and safety that the Koranic Lex can transmit to the Muslim people, may create, at least at the beginning of psychoanalytical work, heavy resistance. (Saegesser, B.: in: Jahrbuch für Kinder- und Jugendlichen Psychoanalyse, 2015–2019. Brandes und Apsel. Frankfurt am Main. Bibliography.) Naturally in our work and life, we always have to do with resistances, but those resistances are very difficult and somehow stony. Patients are not willing to talk about their suffering. They are obliged to *remain silent*. Perhaps this religious-based "resistance" can be transformed, perhaps not, because of their stony or even rocky composition and core.

To close, I write down again the very important scale of personal conduct worth in an Eastern African family structure: the narcissistic and power weight of the family members is in a fundamental way different; most value comes to the commanding and conducting man and his sons. Much less value or importance goes to the woman, wife, mother, and her daughters.

References

Bion, W. R. (2005a). *The Tavistock seminars*. London: Karnac Books.
Bion, W. R. (2005b). *The Italian seminars*. London: Karnac Books.

Hirsi Ali, A. (2015). *Reformiert euch! Warum der Islam sich ändern muss*. München: Albrecht Knaus Verlag.

Koopmans, R. (2019). *Das verfallene Haus des Islam*. München: Verlag C. H. Beck.

Leiris, M. (1985). *Phantom Afrika. Tagebuch einer Expedition von Dakar nach Dschibuti 1931–1933. Erster und zweiter Teil 1985. (Suhrkamp Frankfurt a. M.) TB*. Einleitung: Hans Jürgen Heinrich. Übersetzung: Rolf Wintermeyer. Fortan zitiert als PHA

Özdaglar, A. (2016). *Psychoanalytische Autorität in der Arbeit mit Patienten aus dem muslimischen Kulturkreis*. Brussels: EPF Konferenz.

Quinodoz, D. (2002). *Des mots qui touchent*. Paris: PUF.

Racamier, P.-C. (1993). *Le psychanalyste sans divan*. Paris: Bibliothèque Scientifique Payot.

Saegesser, B. (2012). *Meine psychoanalytische Arbeit in verschiedenen Afrikanischen Ländern*. Basel: Vortrag Psychoanalytisches Seminar.

Saegesser, B. (2014). Psychoanalytische Arbeit mit BB's, Kleinkindern und Müttern in unterschiedlichen afrikanischen Ländern (Le travail psychanalytique avec les bébés, des petits enfants et des mères dans divers pays d'Afrique). *Bulletin No 77. Schweizerische Gesellschaft für Psychoanalyse (SGPsa)*

Saegesser, B. (2015). *Psychoanalytische Feldarbeit in ostafrikanischen Städten I* (P. Bründl, C. E. Scheidt, Jahrbuch der Kinder- und Jugendlichen-Psychoanalyse, Hrsg.) (Bd. 4., S. 211–238). Frankfurt: Brandes und Apsel.

Saegesser, B. (2016a). *Psychoanalytische Feldarbeit in Ostafrikanischen Städten II. Elternschaft in ostafrikanischen Städten* (P. Bründl, C. E. Scheidt, Jahrbuch der Kinder- und Jugendlichen-Psychoanalyse, Hrsg.) (Bd. 5., S. 269–279). Frankfurt: Brandes und Apsel.

Saegesser, B. (2016b). Un travail psychothérapeutique en marge de ma practique psychanalytique et de la culture islamique dans des villes d'Afrique de l' est. Traduction et adaptation de mon manuscripte originale écrit en allemand. Lausanne. *Tribune Psychanalytique, 13.*

Saegesser, B. (2016c). *Eine Skizze psychoanalytischer Arbeit in ostafrikanischen islamischen Städten*. Islamische religiös-weltliche Gesetze und Normen als Basis für Widerstand und Abwehrbewegungen von Patientinnen im Rahmen (situativ angepasster) psychoanalytischer Arbeit. Zürich: "A jour" 2.

Saegesser, B. (2017). *Psychoanalytische Feldarbeit in ostafrikanischen Städten III. Abklärung – Diagnose – Fallbeschreibung. Forschung und Behandlungsplan. Jahrbuch der Kinder- und Jugendlichen-Psychoanalyse* (Peter Bründl und Fernanda Pedrina, Hrsg.) (Bd. 6). Frankfurt: Brandes und Apsel.

Saegesser, B. (2018). *Psychosomatische Prozesse. Jahrbuch der Kinder- und Jugendlichen-Psychoanalyse* (Peter Bründl und Carl Eduard Scheid, Hrsg.) (Bd. 7, S. 198–217). Frankfurt: Branes and Apsel.

Saegesser, B. (2019a). *Geschlechterdifferenz im Spielraum. Jahrbuch der inder- und Jugendlichen-Pychoanalyse* (Peter Bruendl und Helene Timmermann, Hrsg.) (Bd. 8, 254–279). Frankfurt: Branes and Apsel.

Schreiber, C. (1919b). *Kinder des Koran. Was muslimische Schüler lernen*. Berlin: Ullstein.

14 The return of the oppressed, the birth of the other, and collective Western guilt

David Morgan

Paper

The Caterpillar and Alice looked at each other for some time in silence: at last the Caterpillar took the hookah out of its mouth and addressed her in a languid, sleepy voice.

"Who are you?" said the Caterpillar.

This was not an encouraging opening for a conversation. Alice replied, rather shyly, "I – I hardly know, sir, just at present – at least I know who I WAS when I got up this morning, but I think I must have been changed several times since then."

Melanie Klein wrote about the unconscious struggle regarding issues of love, hate, and knowledge. Who we are depends upon the conflicts of love and hate shaped by feelings of knowing or not knowing the primary other and of feeling unknown or negatively known by the other.

Learning and change are impacted by issues of love and hate; what we know or find out about the self and other can generate greater degrees of love or hate. Thus, projective cycles of healthy learning, loving, and growth emerge. Or, in many cases of psychological disorder, a confining cycle of persecution, loss, and censored thought solidify.

To risk a change in how one lives life and how one relates to self and other is often balanced upon how loyal one is to old regimes. To move past these to unknown objective relational connections that break apart the familiar projective identification attachments can be felt as abandonment, loss, betrayal, or guilt instead of being welcomed as independence.

For analytic treatment to be successful, therapists must be constantly working to understand this and interpret this in terms of both defence and underlying anxiety. I would add that analysts' own sense of security in their own certainties at these times, faced with moral political and social uncertainty, must also be faced.

Psychoanalysts are often white middle class.

I have been amused when colleagues living and working from £5 million houses evinced surprise at the intense envy of their patients, when interpretation suggesting that the patient feels the analyst's standard of

DOI: 10.4324/9781003203223-16

living makes it hard for them to feel that they could possibly understand their experiences.

I have said to my patients, at times they are anxious that my theories, my sense of my own certainties and values, are more important to me than they are.

This quest for an open mind is in part based in a belief that others might serve as collateral to find the antidote to fundamental anxiety and mental distress, and projective identification becomes the singular vehicle in a desperate and aggressive hunt for reassurance of meaning and existence.

When projective identification predominates, others become mere extensions of self. They are sources of needed love that are always out of reach, and the focus is more on self-survival and extremes of love and hate than the more object-related, flexible state of mind (Bell, 1996).

I will illustrate how countertransference was useful in becoming aware of certain restricted states of psychic experience and certain un-contained psychological processes that were created by projective dynamics. These particular projective identification mechanisms also provide a very rudimentary or primitive psychic shelter for patients to function without collapsing into internal disintegration. This psychic shelter is experienced as the last refuge of inner security and is felt to be vital, a sanctuary that would be dangerous or psychologically lethal to step out of.

Typical countertransference reactions in the analyst tend to be a give in and join the psychic shelter reaction or become a threatening object trying to forcibly evict the patient from this place of safety.

My first experience of working with a former refugee in an NHS setting included the repeated enquiry or sometime cry: "who are you, what do you do, where do you live?"

The question "who are you?" destabilises and communicates questions of identity into the mind of the analyst as to whether he has the equipment to manage a sense of insecurity and homelessness. When working with people from these situations, it is necessary to be explored in this destabilised state.

The use of projective identification to evacuate knowingly or unknowingly into the other all we do not want to know in ourselves. In us it's our knowledge of our own state's economic exploitation and relative ignorance of the other. Our culture has an ignoble history, and we ourselves in our consulting rooms meeting the other are redolent with that history.

Crucial here are those social processes that support denial of our nature and splitting off uncomfortable aspects of ourselves and locating them in others.

The Nazi regime both created a terror in the entire population of being superfluous and provided people – Jews, gypsies, homosexuals, and so on – who came to embody that superfluousness. "It is they who are superfluous – not me," while believing they were the master race.

The discourse on immigrants and asylum seekers follows a similar logic. We are all anxious about our place in the world; increasingly, we fear being surplus. The refugee threatens us with the fear that there is not enough to go around.

Asylum seekers serve as a projective object, and we can dispose of this unhappy insight. Superfluousness is mixed with racism, and this kind of projective process has a self-amplifying effect – for repositories of projective systems then materialise in our world as a kind of plague, threatening us with what we have disowned.

In our work with asylum seekers, we flounder together in the confusing experiences of difference; I return to their perennial question – "who are you?" I might, however, reply that it's reasonable for them to be interested in me: who am I? Where do I come from? But it's their origins and who they are and how they came here to be in this place is what we are here to think about.

In a first consultation to a hostel for refugees there was no room for my large group to meet. Perhaps a palpable sense of homelessness being put into me?

The people I see often present having been driven to madness or some form of enactment.

I saw someone in prison who had been committed for not allowing the residents in his block of flats into the lift. It seemed that this man was driven to distraction by his own precarious existence and was driven to communicate this feeling through a powerful projection of homelessness into others. It was the other who was temporarily unhoused.

I will illustrate this experience with a few case studies.

Ms C was a 25-year-old woman from Nigeria. She was admitted to the hospital where I acted as a consultant of a clinical supervision group for clinical staff. She had been diagnosed as psychotic – her presenting symptom was a desire to run up to complete strangers in the street and embrace them in a large bear hug. She often chose old women who appeared lonely who were then obviously traumatised by this unprovoked gesture of familiarity.

Ms C's history was that she had been on a student visa studying law with the intent of earning her living as a lawyer. She had, however, failed her exams and been expelled from her course. Her family had hoped that she would be able to send money home after she qualified, and it was clear that they had been very disappointed. It meant that Ms C felt ashamed and expelled from her family. It seemed clear to me that she was reversing her own painful experience of failure and rejection by projecting them onto the aged women whom she embraced as if they were indeed her long-lost relatives whom she felt so excommunicated from.

I was able to share this with staff who found this explanation of her symptoms helpful. However, unfortunately, I forgot to underline how important it was that this thinking was something to be kept in mind rather than directly communicated to the patient. It was, and the patient seemed momentarily to be helped by the link to her own feelings of loss – loss of family, loss of country, and loss of career. That night she managed to break into a senior hospital manager's house in the hospital grounds. He woke up to find her standing over him just looking at him. Of course, he was extremely shocked by this night apparition. I realised that the patient had also been shocked by the clinical insight that she was unprepared to receive. She had fallen back by escalating her previous ways of managing by projecting her feelings onto someone else, and it was they who were shocked and temporally unhinged by her breaking into their home.

Clearly, my failing was to underestimate the importance of ensuring that Ms C's homelessness and alienation were addressed; she overcome her own homelessness by choosing to see others as having need of her company.

I think I have been better able to appreciate how difficult it is for those managing in foreign environments to feel safe enough to do analytic work. I might not have any insight into how frightening it is to be in a foreign culture as I am relatively at home here.

The psychological impact of migration, leaving or entering a country, and the internal experience involves massive psychological struggles and catastrophic change. These tap into the deepest psychotic anxieties.

All this involves learning to adjust and getting accustomed to the rules that govern external life in the new land.

Winnicott (1966) states that, in order to have an integrated sense of self, we need to have an experience of continuity of being.

This term refers to a sense of consistency and internal security that we partially achieve through "environmental validation," which is provided by the continuous interaction between the spatial, temporal, and social dimensions of life (Winnicott, 1966). This means that when what is reflected to us is unfamiliar, we lose a sense of ourselves.

These catastrophic changes lead people to decide to hold on to concrete objects from their original cultures that are imbued with personal symbolic meaning that will help them keep a sense of sameness. This is why it doesn't work when we try to encourage too much assimilation, through the banning of religious dress. For the immigrant, it's a way of retaining contact with the old regime.

Mr A was young man from the Middle East who had been in analysis for a few years. His visa was running out, but he had an urgent problem. He came from a relatively orthodox family. His original reason for seeking treatment was his inability to make and sustain relationships with women, any women. He was 33 years of age and had not managed any sexual relationships. The problem seemed to have its roots in a very strong oedipal attachment to his mother to the point that she seemed to undermine any possibility of another woman. There was a strong ethical prohibition to sex before marriage from his religious orthodoxy, and Mr A seemed unable to separate from what seemed to be a rather infantilising mother.

He used to wish that his parents would help him select his wife as many of his friend's parents had done for their sons. But he also somehow felt he should be able to do this for himself – something he put down to his ethnically diverse schooling and the influence of his peers.

In his background, up until his generation, it had been the norm for parents or matchmakers to do the arranging.

As Mr A.'s treatment progressed, he began to meet women via an ethnically focused dating site. He faced the threat of deportation. He was able to explore his sexuality and eventually met his wife independently. She was someone who was not from an orthodox background but attended what seemed to be a very liberal place of worship and was from a family who seemed more interested in the symbolic manifestations of their rich heritage than the more concrete, more fundamental interpretation of religious texts.

Looking back, I do wonder how much my unconscious influence, with my ostensibly liberal values and non-religious background, may have encouraged this development.

This conflict between different value systems, his wife's and maybe his analyst's, came to a head later on in his treatment. He married this more liberal girlfriend, and within a year, they gave birth to a male baby.

In his analysis, he explored the issue of being a father and how much he wanted his son to adopt his religious and ethnic background. He had by this time, in fact from the first month when I betrayed my ignorance of holy days, realised that I was not from their ethnic descent. We had explored throughout his analysis how my ignorance of his ethnicity was both a hindrance and, in some less obvious ways, an advantage. Indeed, I have observed that many orthodox patients prefer an apparently irreligious analyst to someone from their own background.

It inevitably came to pass that the question of circumcision became prominent. He was in no doubt that he would follow tradition and would have his son circumcised. However, his wife was very concerned about the procedure, as she knew of a friend whose son had had complications following the ceremony. In my countertransference, I struggled with my own views – for example, that it was an anachronism, from desert cultures, and I knew friends, mainly psychoanalysts, who had undergone this procedure despite cultural expectations. Other friends told me of the dis-identification from the father that non-circumcision represented and how non-circumcised boys from Jewish and Muslim backgrounds often felt alienated. One story, probably apocryphal, told of children trying to perform their own ritual; so desperate were they to "fit in."

I also wondered why anyone should listen to these mad old prophets and the immense need to belong to fear punishment for forsaking the father. While I still wonder why anyone should go along unthinkingly with the words of these "prophets," I do wonder if there is also a real price to be paid by those who don't.

Helping the patient think for himself was threatened by my own prejudices, however rational I thought I was being. My supervisor surprised me by stating that there was no issue, because, of course, it should be done. This surprised me, as until then everything had been transference based in this supervision, but this issue seemed to be beyond psychoanalytic theorising. I have always been surprised at how a number of my colleagues have maintained strong religious beliefs during their training and careers.

With Mr A, a number of issues soon came into the analysis when he helpfully brought a dream. In the dream, he was standing on a station platform, and two trains arrived simultaneously – one was going to Hendon and the other to Hampstead. His associations were that Hendon clearly represented his orthodoxy and Hampstead the home of psychoanalysis. He felt that "he was on the horns of a dilemma" in that he both wanted to be liberal minded and, at the same time, follow his conscience in relation to his ethnic traditions.

I interpreted that it was important for him that I was able to help him think about decisions like his son's circumcision. The question he posed was, am I able to help him have a mind of his own rather than feel he has to obey orthodoxies including mine? Of course, this interpretation was redolent with my own belief system, but as an analyst, how could it not be? Did it help enable my patient simply to think for himself, or was it promoting the idea that having a mind of his own was more important than his rooted-ness in the ancient value systems based on his ethnic traditional values?

The very practice of analysis flies in the face of orthodoxies and fundamentalist thinking, yet clearly it can become dominated by certainties itself.

After a few weeks, the patient decided that he would go ahead with the religious celebration of circumcision. I did feel that the religious value system had exerted its power over him, and yet it was right for this patient to submit, as I saw it, or assert his right to pursue his own direction independent of me, as he saw it. In the exploration of the dream, I felt there was a struggle for shared ground where two minds and ideas could be considered. The station at least represented a place where choices could be made; the patient's apparent borderline condition, where he was stuck on the platform unable to decide was precisely what his background was unable to equip him with – the capacity to bear uncertainty. It is of interest to note that at the actual ceremony he had been able to contain his mother, who in an attempt to upstage proceedings and rival the baby got into an argument with the mother-in-law. The patient was able to stand up to his mother pointing out her upstaging of proceedings in a way that she was able to respond to. I felt our exploration of mutual space had allowed something new to happen in the family dynamic.

In my countertransference replete with cultural normative values I would have to admit that I found the idea of circumcising a small baby disturbing. I had to struggle with and help my patient feel there was space to think with me. I therefore had to struggle with my orthodoxy based on my experience rather than impose it on him. I think this exploration allowed him to decide for himself but enabled him to stand up to his mother's domination.

My disturbance over difference eventually gave way to space to think.

Ms B was in her 40s; she was single with two children and from an African background. She was someone who had come to England ten years before I saw her. Her presenting problem was a need to control her anger – particularly towards Caucasian men. In one case she had "frighteningly lost control" by attacking a taxi after its driver had mistaken her for a prostitute while walking in the north London suburb where she lived. This reprisal on her part seemed reasonable on the one hand, but on the other, her preoccupation and sense of grievance with this tendency in some racist British men left her concerned that one day she would get hurt.

From the beginning Ms B criticised me for being a white male. The fact she said that I was evidently Welsh did not in any way mean that I did not represent a section of British colonialist attitudes that had enslaved her country of origin. How could I, she said, hope to understand her experience when our experiences, both racial and gender based were so opposite? I said that I thought she was right to explore with me what sort of analyst I was and whether I had any equipment that could be used to understand her. It was possible that I did not – indeed she doubted any white man's capacity to truly understand. I said it remained to be seen whether she should continue her analysis or end it, because I might be a bigoted racist analyst. She seemed thoughtful about my apparent willingness to be thought about as such an unattractive figure. Clearly, the analytic vehicle I was using so far did not deserve the same fate as the taxi her abuser was driving.

She stayed in analytic therapy with me. It transpired that there was a great deal that I did not understand. She hardly knew her parents and had been brought up by the tribe. She seemed to have many aunts and uncles who looked after her. The lack of any real parental couple meant that it felt, at least to me, that a lot of the usual reference points from her past were lost. Did this mean that this tribe's child-rearing practices left children without a clear sense of a parental couple, or was I pathologising a culture, different to my own experience? In the transference, I experienced a great deal of confusion as to who I was in relation to the patient. It was easy to begin with to believe that this represented the patient's own confusion from her extended family experience: her lack of reference points, as her parents were not the main caregivers. In fact, it transpired that, despite my belief based on a simplistic countertransference response, I almost missed the subtler message, which was "Can you, analyst bear the confusion in your usual reference points, the couple, the oedipal relationship, without reinforcing your position by pushing your idea of normality back into me?"

I saw her for many years, and her tendency to get into fights reduced, as did my wish to impose my belief system onto her. It was this exploration of my fear of loss of purpose – the fear of losing my rootedness in the therapeutic process, as I understood it – that allowed something other than recrimination to develop. This seemed to be what was needed – not my need to reinforce my own experience that her background challenged.

Unlike nuclear families, tribes allow diversification of investment, no foreclosure, more power balance, less competitiveness among siblings, precisely what industrialisation has destroyed, and psychopathology is a by-product of that.

What was abnormal was her no longer being in the tribe or close to the tribe, thus the confusion. I have understood this struggle as akin to the power of nationalism in that when we are under threat, we often look for flags that we can stand under to protect our identity from fragmentation. Psychoanalytic theory can also be used this way when patients bring "foreign" experiences into the consulting room – it functions as a form of protection to the analyst whose own normative experiences are put to the test.

It is enormously important for the analyst to be discovered as someone who might be able to think about their own restricted experience without using psychoanalytic theory defensively as a psychic retreat.

This defensive retreat can include the reduction of ethnic beliefs to psychotic mechanisms, the issue of sexual difference to failures in oedipal development, or other forms of reductionism.

This is the difficult task but maybe the only experience some of our patients have ever had of diverse thinking. A vital part of this process seems to be aware of the initial impulses in the countertransference to repudiate alien experiences as pathologies.

Therapeutic work also has an important preventive function, since traumatic internal experiences that are not worked through may lead to acting-outs, enactments, and intergenerational trauma, affecting the next generations.

Socially and politically what can we do?

States have the right to meaningful borders; the problem created by capital on the one hand, climate change on the other, leads to increased competition for resources that immigration can bring.

Western policy towards refugees over the last decades needs rethinking: the economic relationship between richer and poorer countries using migrants as economic "ferrymen" to carry money and energy and ideas between the two worlds, much more equally in both directions than currently, and with far greater government assistance (Grinberg & Grinberg, 2004).

The experience of otherness is, as we all know, threatening. It can be uncomfortable facing what is not familiar or getting close to something different. Rejecting what is foreign may be just another expression of our attempt to maintain our "continuity of being" – searching for reassurances that reflect only that which we can identify with or relate to. (Berger 2008).

This illustrates how careful we have to be in our practices to bear the challenge to our norms that differences confront us with.

Psychoanalytic thinking needs to be able to wrestle with these prejudices if our current world situation, which has created refugees, is to be addressed. In particular, how can psychoanalysis help us to understand the powerful's imperviousness to the injury they cause to others, and what psychic structure enables the powerful to obviate evidence of the harm they/we cause?

References

Bell, D. (1996). The primitive mind of state. *Psychoanalytic Psychotherapy*, 10(1), 45–57.

Berger, J. (2008). *In hold everything dear. Dispatches on survival and resistance*. London: Verso Press.

Grinberg, L., & Grinberg, R. (2004). Psychoanalytic perspectives on migration. In D. Bell (Ed.), *Psychoanalysis and culture: A Kleinian perspective* (pp. 154–169). Great Britain: Karnac Books.

Winnicott, D. (1966). The location of cultural experience. *The International Journal of Psychoanalysis*, 48(3), 368–372.

15 Trauma, refugees, and ethnopsychoanalytical experiences

Maya Nadig

1 Transcultural Communication

When members of two cultures meet, each has a specific perspective of the other, shaped by conscious and unconscious personal experiences and by the beliefs and values of their own milieu of belonging as well as by the views held there on the other's culture. However, there is not only one fixed image about the other person, but depending on the situation, a very complex dynamic unfolds immediately.

Therapeutic or counselling encounters are based on the desire to understand and to be understood by each other what creates a shared space that incorporates elements from both cultures. It's a kind of transitional or in-between space in which both participants relate to each other but maintain their personal view from outside of what is happening – that is, a third reflective position. So far, similarities and strangeness are simultaneously present and negotiated. Both the therapist and his counterpart are in contact with each other and oscillate between their associations, personal sensations for the other, discomfort and their foreboding anxieties that arise while their unconscious perceives more than they "know." Gradually, in such a tense and ambivalent "professional" and individual approach, defence mechanisms emerge to manage the unease and confusion. We could say that "transcultural situations" involve a historical and current blurring of perceived differences and supposed boundaries. But often, beyond the differences, common connections, interdependencies, and protective and structuring mechanisms of protection emerge and also shape the contact.

2 Ethnopsychoanalytic Research with the Mosuo

Between 2010 and 2019, I made six visits to the Mosuo, a matrilineal society in Southern China bordering Tibet and at the edge of the Himalayas. The Mosuo do not practice marriage. The love relationships are open, sometimes changeable, and take the form of nightly visits by the

DOI: 10.4324/9781003203223-17

man to the woman's courtyard. The children remain with their mother's extended family and their blood relatives throughout their lives. I was fascinated, but also shocked, on my first visit that the family members who tend and carry babies around, cradle or shake them, but barely make eye contact with them. They pass it immediately to another family member if the little one becomes uncomfortable. I was surprised and disturbed and wondered if this was preparation for the open love relationships that do not require the children's fathers to perform duties that arise from fatherhood.

The children always belong to the household of the woman who cares for them, including the mother's brother or uncle. The fathers are insignificant. (Shih, 2010; Yang & Mathieu, 2004)

We, a psychoanalytic colleague who visited me during my third stay, and I came up with the idea that these may be immature and superficial forms of relationships and that the absence of the father has negative consequences for the lives of the adults and children. The avoidance of individual and deeper contact between the partners and between mother and baby probably represented an inability to perceive and acknowledge the differentiated emotions of the other and consequently to provide an adequate response to the child. The effect on the child would be similar to that of a depressed and unavailable, early "dead" mother according to A. Green (1986) and Stern (1998). We suspected that this would lead to relationship dysfunction, aggression suppression, later depression, and lack of deep bonding. This concept allowed us to accommodate our discomfort and fascination with the loneliness and the changing love relationships. There was the feeling that perhaps one had found an interesting research result. One could, if one wished, quickly publish articles and give lectures about it. Fortunately, during my further visits I was able to verify my doubts about our psychoanalytic concept and understood that it was partly pejorative, arrogant, and not adequate.

In Mosuo culture, the matrilineal family is of utmost importance. The close cohesion of the large group ensured their survival at an altitude of 3,000 metres amidst threats from raids by the Chinese dynasties, who needed slaves and soldiers, and the warlike Yi, who lived in large numbers around them and readily robbed Mosuo women as slaves and wives. The socialisation of the children is done through intensive and reliable physical affection and reassurance by changing family members rather than through individual contact and deepening of the individual relationship. As a result, the family group becomes their internal object. Accordingly, the mother hands the child over to the care of the family group about one month after birth and has only reduced contact with him, especially during breastfeeding in the first year (Cai, 2001; Coler, 2005; Knödel, 1995; Nadig, 2013).

What can be observed?

- The mother withdraws from the baby after one month. She goes to the field in the day and breastfeeds at lunch and in the evening. She works in the fields and breastfeeds at lunch and in the evening. The shared delights of breastfeeding and tenderness seem to be suppressed and with them the arousal of the erogenous zones from which pleasurable sensuality and sexuality develop. Does this prevention of closeness and intimacy interrupt and keep in check incestuous desires in the close family structure?
- The relatives do not establish a personal intimate relationship with the baby to examine his specific motivation for restlessness and individual current feelings. It seems that only the external restlessness and physical movements are observed and reassured, but no conclusions are drawn about his internal states.
- In fact, interruptions of the baby's expressions occur. At the same time, however, there is an absolutely reliable group that lovingly takes the child in its arms, reassures it, and involves it. When it is very tired, it comes on the back very close to the body of grandmother, aunt, uncle, and so on.
- The frequent change of persons between the family members possibly means a permanent stimulation that prevents mentalisation of the internal, individual states and contains the message not to pay attention to them. Can this also keep libidinous impulses flat and prevent incestuous desires?
- Group membership and identity are of central importance. Being reliably held on the "group arm" has other consequences than holding with us: namely, a strong attachment to all members of the group. It prevents "individualistic excesses" such as a one-sided mother or uncle bond that could disturb the balance of the group (Nadig, 2014a).

This way of dealing with the baby also has something to do with the management of emotional relations in the matrilineal extended household, to which children remain attached throughout their lives, living in close quarters with mother, aunts and uncles, grandmother and their siblings, cousins, and other relatives. Can this lifelong closeness in the extended family be balanced by the simultaneous keeping of distance and the avoidance of closeness and separation? Thus, in comparison to Western nuclear families, different psychological structures and bonds between individuals emerge in the matrilineal household. Does this result in a kind of impoverishment of cathexis, as André Green (1986) describes it? No. Group-based socialisation produces consistent physical familiarity with almost all family members without giving too much emphasis to personal desires and attachments.

3 Distorted Perception and Reflection

The methodological approaches of ethnological field research and psychoanalytical research of the unconscious show a strong affinity. In both disciplines, the scientific exploration of the unknown is an intense social endeavour, itself subject to social conditions and dependencies as well as to the subjectivity of the researcher. Ethnological fieldwork is a dynamic technique of qualitative research: similar to psychoanalytic research about the unconscious, it draws its insights from encounters with people from other milieus or cultures and from relations with them. These encounters often trigger alienation and uncertainty. Clarifying self-reflection could mediate between the social field and science by exposing reductionist categories from one's own culture that structure field notes or case presentations such as ethnocentric or moralistic evaluation or psychoanalytic terms in the style of wild interpretations, and so on.

The "Ethnopsychoanalytic Workshop of Interpretation" (Nadig, 2009, 2014b), which I developed and conducted at the University of Bremen tries to interpret transcultural encounters to understand the psychodynamic. In group sessions with students and postgraduates we focused on the social dynamics that evolved in a transcultural research situation. The aim is to work with the unconscious parts in the presented ethnological research notes, which contain in their original form the unconscious transcultural dynamics that developed during the field research: for example, transference, countertransference, resistance of the researcher or ethnocentric projections and attributions on both sides, and so on.

Postcolonial theories of culture similarly understand culture as a process of encounter, engagement, and intersection with other cultures (Clifford & Marcus, 1986; Geertz, 1973; Fuchs & Berg, 1993; Hall, 1996a, 1996b; Robinow, 2007). A categorising and valuating view of culture is always attributive and projective. We need to be aware of the discourse we hear publicly about immigrants in political, media, and everyday discussions and the impact it has on the treatment they receive. It must be remembered that researchers, therapists, and counsellors are also themselves part of this public opinion and the implicit prejudices and discourses of their culture (Abu Lughod, 2006). But beyond the differences, in ethnological encounters emerge and grow personal contacts, common connections, dependencies, and mechanisms of mutual protection.

When working with refugees and migrants, a similar transcultural tension emerges. We can better understand them by considering, for example, the forms of discrimination and exclusion they experience through our culture, and also by considering those complex medial and symbolic mechanisms that influence who belongs to a society. The search for the mechanisms of social exclusion shifts the focus away from the conspicuous behaviour of the culturally other to the social structures that surround and define them here.

An Israeli therapist writes about her life in Frankfurt:

> The fact that I am Israeli and Jewish comes to the fore in conversation with people living here, and not me as a person. That only comes to the fore secondarily. . . . What bothers me personally most in Germany – to exaggerate – is that I am not seen as a personality, but as a symbol for something. . . . The dominant feeling for me as a foreigner was to be constantly misunderstood.
>
> (76)

The author wonders if she really understands what the other person is trying to say and if he understands what she means. She describes a projection of one's own generalised images and values onto the national and cultural other. In this way, the internal diversities of a nation and its cultures are unified and discursively annihilated and dehumanised (ben Kalifa-Schor, 1998).

Our fears and defences sometimes make it difficult for us to communicate undistortedly with others or strangers. Unconscious ambivalences and conflicts with the stranger risk a splitting of our negative "bad" parts and their projection onto them. Admittedly, this relieves us for the moment. But the splitting excludes undesired parts from the psychic development and maturation; in this way they are put on ice, so to speak. The therapist will not have enough possibilities for reflection and a playful handling of his irritations. His projection makes empathy and compassion impossible, and the therapeutic process threatens to freeze. Under this condition, the desire to understand the other may cause anxiety. The inner conflict consists now between keeping on the projection or withdrawing it and perceiving one's own inner conflicts. The withdrawal of the projection is a prerequisite for being able to encounter the stranger in an unprejudiced way (Erdheim, 2002).

A related form of projective dealing with the fear of the alien consists in the development of theoretical categories and methodological procedures towards the other. The ethnopsychoanalyst Georges Devereux, in his book *From Anxiety to Methods* (1967), advocates a psychoanalytically based critique of strictly applied objective methods and scientistic approaches to the object of research. He believes that an encounter with foreign people and their worlds almost always triggers fear in scientists, ethnologists, and therapists and that unconscious defence mechanisms such as repression, splitting, denial, idealisation, devaluation, projection, and so on are used against it. In science, the implementation of these defence mechanisms usually happens in the context of the chosen categorising methods and theories. Technical measuring methods, quantitative questionnaires, "clear" hypotheses, and behavioural instructions, as well as assigning the foreign behaviour into scientific categories create a distance of the researcher/therapist to his subject/counterpart. This links him again more strongly to his own cultural basis of thinking and alleviates his restlessness and uncertainty.

4 "Trauma" and Homelessness

However, it is not only the culturally strange that we encounter in therapy and counselling sessions, but we also easily experience the psychologically strange as unbearable. Many refugees and migrants bring with them psychological injuries that are difficult to access and endure. These also seem heavy and burdensome to us and are easily wrapped up in preconceived notions.

Sverre Varvin, for instance, writes about our relationship to refugees under the title: *Between Compassion and Dehumanization*: "When xenophobia becomes part of the political or religious narrative, and serves to fuel conflict between groups, unconscious processes at both the individual and group levels are set in motion" (Varvin, 2018, p. 199).

In contact with and in the discourse about strangers, one's own unconscious conflicts – such as sibling rivalry, experiences of deprivation, separation, and individuation – are activated. The split between "good" and "bad" and between libidinous and aggressive strivings lead to projections of one's own undesirable parts into the discourse field about refugees and migrants.

He traces the fate of the concept of trauma in the discourse of therapists working with refugees and connects it with the confusing and elusive psychodynamics of trauma: this is dissociated and cannot be symbolised psychologically. That means that the trauma cannot find a language. It triggers psychological and physical pain, depression, confusion, panic, breakdowns. The therapist is at times drawn into the patient's non-symbolised, fragmentary scenes. The therapist can provide a holding, containing framework under the condition that he can get involved in the patient's fragmented non-symbolised manifestations. "This means that the analyst (therapist, counselor) must accept that he lives with the patient in realms of self-awareness and memory that are agonizingly meaningless and at times a single horror" (ibid. 208). He experiences an absolute helplessness in the face of these manifestations and seeks to escape this helplessness by attaching the label "trauma" to the other person. The concept may provide clinicians and therapists with some relief from the unbearable feelings evoked by these extreme experiences. "Traumatization implies an extreme encounter with primal fears; and the relationship with a traumatized person might bring up similar anxieties (in the therapist)" (ibid 211).

Varvin writes convincingly:

> The term "trauma" then becomes a place where very remote and intolerable elements can be deposited, so that something like meaning

can be assigned to the uncanny as it is aroused in countertransference. This emptying of the concept suggests that "trauma" is often used as an object of projection for uncanny fantasies and feelings. Trauma now stands for a territory of extreme fear, destructiveness, and a perverted Eros.

(ibid 210)

The use of certain diagnostic terms as empty shells creates a desired distance between the traumatised person and the caregiver/therapist. However, this denies the other fundamentally human qualities. The therapist's reification of trauma serves to reduce his own anxiety and reifies the other.

But there is a further difficult problem: many refugees and migrants bring with them further psychological injuries that are difficult to access and endure. Their complaints such as sleeplessness, forgetfulness, apathy, and so on conceal often a deep feeling of loss and forlornness that contains a double homelessness: an easily recognisable homelessness connected with the flight on the one hand and a homelessness stemming from childhood and connected with the object relations of that time on the other. In the "early homelessness" we encounter another nameless injury, also foreign in appearance, which renders us helpless and is often difficult to recognise and endure. Joshua Durban (2019) describes homelessness, this "being nowhere" as an early childhood experience that later in adult life can be emotionally activated like a not-symbolised trauma when changing country or milieu. Early homelessness arises from disruptions, separations, and disasters in early childhood where no secure sense of being-in-the-world could be found, and this is not necessarily connected with migration. Durban describes the construction of a sense of home as a complex achievement involving three components: first, being safely at home in the body-as-mother (constitution) and second, internalising the mother-as-me, which means creating an inner and an interpersonal space. These two levels finally enable the development of the third level: a triangular oedipal space. The complicated construction of an inner home that emerges in the interplay between these elements is accompanied by pronounced anxieties, conflicts, and unconscious fantasies. Disturbances in this process can lead to severe pathologies that emerge together with paranoid-schizoid anxieties, which in the case of "early homelessness" are directed against closer relationships and the dangers, gains, losses that accompany them. In the case of this "being nowhere," as Durban calls it, a kind of self-dissection or autistic encapsulation defends against the feeling of falling, having no skin, losing orientation, dissolving.

In the low-frequency therapies with refugees at the Center for Intercultural Psychiatry and Psychotherapy at the Charité Hospital, I have often experienced how complex and confusing the interweaving of more recent injuries from war and flight with very early experiences of neglect, violence in the family, of catastrophes in the environment is sensed by the therapist. Early abandonment and disruption of the primary relationship are connected with existential and "nameless fears" (Bion) which are frightening and difficult to bear for the counsellor/analyst. Getting on the same level with the patient, the therapist comes in touch with the nameless fears, absorbs them, and feels their existential quality. Then the patient can begin to incorporate and internalise the analyst as a good, constant, and living "home-object."

5 Example from an Analysis

In the analysis with a young Kurdish man who was politically persecuted in Turkey, a double traumatisation gradually emerged: on the one hand as a persecuted student in political opposition and on the other hand "behind" his homelessness in early childhood when his father died and his mother disappeared in deep depression. After a suicide attempt, he came severely depressed from the clinic to me at the age of 33, appearing as some years younger.

He had absolved academic studies and spoke German and English very well. As the youngest of seven children, he had been living in Germany, since three years in the house of his older brother and his family, who had also emigrated and worked in a restaurant.

In our analysis, he talked very distantly and with long silences about his actual life. Sometimes he would fall into a speech breakdown and a half sleep, seeing dreamlike images and scenes – pictures of his childhood. The patient's silence, speech breakdown, and lack of emotion caused intense feelings of powerlessness and pain in me.

I always had to cope anew with the fact that I did not know the patient's traumatic experiences and could not understand what happened in him. But I felt a strong need to let and accept him without urging with interpretations. Mostly I felt like holding him just as he was. Since he came regularly, I knew he could use our sessions three times a week.

When he began to relate more concrete scenes from his actual life, I began to understand his deep inner loneliness. His tellings of the control his brothers exerted on him, their misuse of his intellectual capacities, and his permanent disappointment that ended in terrible depressive states triggered in my feelings impotence and anger that were hard to bear. I began to understand that underneath the trauma of political persecution as a student – he was arrested and subjected to a mock shooting – and his flight to Germany, he suffered from early childhood traumatisation and homelessness. The death of the father six months after his birth left his mother alone with seven kids exposed to the interests and power strategies of the family clan. While she did not agree to get married as second wife with one of the brothers of her passed-away husband, the clan isolated her with the children. They were very poor, and all of them had to work hard in the fields to get enough to eat. He spoke without emotions about different situations at that time as if they were "short stories." The concrete happenings were embedded into the wider context in which they happened: the village, the year, the power relations, the common rituals, the relatives. In this form he related the desperation and the courageous fight of his mother or the nearly sadistic negation of the relatives to help them; a visit of the uncle who was a writer and lived in Switzerland and talked with him; that the brothers cheated him, taking the best part of something or in a situation; and so on. I realised more and more the efforts and pains of himself and the brothers working in the fields before and after school or bringing up a newborn calf until it could be sold for good money. Then the loss of the home village when he was 13, and the mother deciding to move to Ankara because there were more possibilities for her growing-up children to earn money. And I felt his terrible isolation and loneliness in the early childhood and in the poor district of the big city, where they fearfully had to maintain the family and learn to speak another language and hide their cultural background.

I understood that in this peasant family's internal cohesion was the highest principle of survival. This was expressed in a strict kinship and age hierarchy. The "little one" always had to obey unconditionally the elder ones and be content with what they left for him. There existed still only one family account for all of them. Every sibling had to give his actual earnings into this common account. But the expenses were managed by the elder brothers. His socialisation, like that of his siblings, was focused exclusively on the preservation of the family group. There was no place for individual needs, relationships, and bonds, except for the bond with the mother, as the head. She bound the children closely to her through guilt-inducing demands and needs. This led him to call her almost daily in Turkey. The inner bond with the next older brother was existentially important for him, because he, more than the mother, gave him the feeling of being somewhat at home and protected in the world. His dependence and powerlessness towards his brother and siblings acted as a blockade against change through psychoanalysis. The permanent contacts among the members assure that the group is functioning and defends its members against danger. Without his group the individual would be lost (cf. Parin, 1978).

Only when I felt and patiently endured his early homelessness in countertransference, did I understand the internal psychic structure of this peasant family and could better accept and address it. Difficult and hurtful memories with his siblings and mother surfaced, and he almost incredulously and astonishingly discovered their "assaults" on him. Now he began to feel his anger and some resistance arose, which he began to gently assert. This enabled him – without breaking with the brother and family – to find and go his own way.

6 Short Summary

Ethnopsychoanalysis and psychoanalysis try to approach the different cultural environments and their people with discretion and caution in order to understand their functioning. General knowledge of the different social structures, their history, and their economic foundations is a good prerequisite for approaching the socialisation and attitudes of people in this society. However, the quick application of psychoanalytic categories in contact with people from other cultures can be essentialising. Many of our theories assume a world ordered differently in civil society – a world that has gone through industrial society and now through digitalisation. Our notion of a mature adult is partly linked to defined notions of individuality and autonomy (Dumont, 1991; LeVine, 1998). Some psychoanalytical and psychological categories are implicitly built on them. Depending on a specific situation, they often do not do justice to the other, but implicitly devalue him. By a longer process of getting to know, letting oneself be touched by the culturally and psychologically foreign allows psychoanalytic knowledge to become a constructive and understanding tool to comprehend what is happening in the inner and outer world of the counterpart or the patient. In such situations we have to accept that we do not know how does triangulation occur without a father? What does it mean to be carried by the group, to have a so-called group ego? Challenging questions and perspectives come up that partly relativise our categories. And then it gets exciting.

References

Abu-Lughod, L. (2006). Writing against culture. In E. Lewin (Ed.), *Feminist anthropology: A reader* (pp. 153–169). Blackwell Publishing Ltd: Malden, MA.

Ben Kalifa-Schor, G. (1998). Interkulturelle Aspekte in der psychoanalytischen Arbeit mit Migranten. In *Analytische Kinder- und Jugendlichen-Psychotherapie* (S. 531–549). Zeitschrift für Theorie und Praxis der Kinder- und Jugendlichen-Psychoanalyse. Heft 100, XXIX. Jg., 4/1998. {Intercultural aspects in psychoanalytic work with migrants.} Frankfurt

Bion, W. R. (1962). *Learning from experience*. London: Heinemann.

Cai, H. (2001). *A society without fathers or husbands: The Na of China*. New York and Cambridge, MA: Zone Books.

Clifford, J., & Marcus, G. (1986). *Writing culture: The poetics and politics of ethnography: A school of American research advanced seminar*. Berkeley, CA and London: University of California Press.

Coler, R. (2005). *El reino de las mujeres: el último matriarcado*. Buenos Aires: Planeta. {The kingdom of women: the last matriarch}

Devereux, G. (1967). *Angst und Methode in den Verhaltenswissenschaften*. München: Carl Hanser Verlag {From anxiety to methods)

Dumont, L. (1991). *Individualismus. Zur Ideologie der Moderne*. Frankfurt/M.: Campus. {Individualism. On the ideology of modernity}

Durban, J. (2019). Heimat, Heimatlosigkeit und Nirgendwosein in der frühen Kindheit. *Psyche, 1*, 17–41. {Home, homelessness, being nowhere in early childhood.}

Erdheim, M. (2002). Verzerrungen des Fremden. In O. Gutjahr (Hg.), *Fremde* (S. 21–46). Würzburg: Königshausen & Neumann. {Distortions of the strange}.

Fuchs, M., & Berg, E. (1993). *Kultur, soziale Praxis, Text: die Krise der ethnographischen Repräsentation*. Frankfurt: Suhrkamp. {Culture, Social Practice, Text: The crisis of the ethnographic representation}

Geertz, C. (1973). *The interpretation of cultures: Selected essays*. New York: Basic Books.

Green, A. (1986) The dead mother. In *A. Green: On private madness* (pp. 142–173). London: Hogarth.

Hall, S. (1996a). Introduction: Who needs 'identity'? In S. Hall & P. du Gay (Hg.), *Questions of cultural identity* (S. 1–17). London: Sage.

Hall, S. (1996b). Politics of identity. In *Terence ranger, yunas samad & ossie stuart: Culture, identity, politics. Ethnic minorities in britain* (pp. 129–135). Aldershot: Averbury.

Knödel, S. (1995). *Die matrilinearen Mosuo von Yongning: eine quellenkritische Auswertung moderner chinesischer Ethnographien*. Münster: Lit., {The matrilineal Mosuo of Yongning: A source-critical evaluation of modern Chinese ethnography.}

LeVine, R., et al. (1998). *Childcare and culture. Lessons from Africa*. Cambridge: Cambridge University Press.

Nadig, M. (2004). Transculturality in progress theoretical and methodological aspects drawn from cultural studies and psychoanalysis. In Hans Jörg Sandkühler & Hong-Bin Lim (Hg.), *Transculturality – epistemology, ethics, and politics* (pp. 9–21). Frankfurt a. M.: Europäischer Verlag der Wissenschaften.

Nadig, M. (2009). Einführung in eine ethnopsychoanalytische Deutungswerkstatt. In G. Schneider & H.-J. Eilts (Hg.), *Klinische Psychoanalyse heute – Forschungsfelder und Perspektiven* (S. 419–426). Frankfurt: DPV-Herbsttagungsband 2008. {Introduction to an ethnopsychoanalytic workshop of interpretation.}

Nadig, M. (2013). Stabilisierung von Kultur – Modulierung von Wandel und Dominanzverhältnissen durch regulierte Ökonomie und Sexualität. Das Beispiel der Mosuo und anderer Gesellschaften. In A. Hepp & A. Lehmann-Wermser (Hg.), *Transformationen des Kulturellen: Prozesse des gegenwärtigen Kulturwandels*. Wiesbaden: Springer VS, (S. 33–56). {Stabilization of culture – modulation of change and relations of dominance through regulated economy and sexuality. The example of the Mosuo and other societies. In A. Hepp & A. Lehmann-Wermser (Eds.), *Transformations of the cultural: Processes of contemporary cultural change.*}

Nadig, M. (2014a). Mütter, Kinder und Verwandte in einer matrilinearen Gesellschaft. In C. Schader (Ed.), *Möslein-Teising: Keine friedfertige Frau*. Giessen: Psychosozial. {Mothers, children and relatives in a matrilineal society. In C. Schader (Ed.), *Möslein-Teising: No peaceable woman.*}

Nadig. M. (2014b). Schreiben über "die" Mosuo. Schwierigkeiten, einer fremden Kultur gerecht zu werden. Ethnopsychoanalytische Überlegungen zur Sozialisation bei den Mosuo in Südchina. In O. Gutjahr (Ed.), *Interkulturalität. Konstruktionen des Anderen. Freiburger literaturpsychologische Gespräche* (Bd. 32). Würzburg: Königshausen & Neumann {Writing about "the" Mosuo. Difficulties in living up to a foreign culture. Ethnopsychoanalytic reflections on socialization among the Mosuo in South China}. In O. Gutjahr (Ed.), *Interculturality. Constructions of the other. Freiburger literaturpsychologische Gespräche* (Vol. 32). Würzburg: König-shausen & Neumann, Frankfurt.

Parin, P. (1978). Aspekte des Gruppen-Ich. In P. Parin (Ed.), *Der Widerspruch im Subjekt. Ethnopsychoanalytische Studien* (pp. 153–174). Frankfurt a. M.: Syndikat. {The contradiction in the subject. Ethnopsychoanalytic Studies}

Rabinow, P. (2007). Anthropological observation and self-formation. In J. Biehl, B. Good, & A. Kleinman (Eds.), *Subjectivity: Ethnographic investigations* (pp. 98–118). Berkeley, CA and London: University of California Press.

Shih, C.-K. (2010). *Quest for harmony: The Moso traditions of sexual union and family life*. Stanford: Stanford University Press.

Stern, D. (1998). *The motherhood constellation*. New York: Basic Books.

Varvin, S. (2018). Über unser Verhältnis zu Flüchtlingen: Zwischen Mitleid und Entmenschlichung. *Psyche, 8*, 194–215. {About our relationship to refugees: Between compassion and dehumanization.}

Yang, E. N., & Mathieu, C. (2004). *Leaving mother lake: A girlhood at the edge of the world*. New York and Boston: Back Bay Books.

Part B

Psychoanalysis and the UN

16 Advocating Psychoanalysis at the UN

Laura Ravaioli

I commit my dream to you
The people have the power.

Patti Smith

In a country where I did not speak the language well enough, I was waiting for the bus to the airport. It was extremely crowded (this happened long before COVID-19 and its restrictions), and with my large luggage, I had the impression that other passengers looked at me with a severe gaze, especially because I did not understand the words of the speaker announcing the next stop, and I had to move to see the screen. After some stops many other people came in, and *I* felt irritated, because in the meanwhile I became a member of the *group of the bus*, feeling then those new passengers were kind of *intruders*. These odd feelings reminded me of the concept of internal racism (Davids, 2011) and made me reflect about the privilege of developing some psychic tools to be aware of it and that belong to our training as psychoanalysts and enrich us as human beings. A similar situation happened during a conference on migration, where several colleagues joined later and caused the complaints of those who were already in the room: the phrase "[N]o one should enter here anymore" reproduced those immigration bans that the conference was exactly discussing.

The mental disposition to self-observation about feelings, thoughts, and behaviours and the attention to group psychodynamics give psychoanalysts the chance to reflect on micro-events like the ones in the bus or at the conference, enlightening some primitive mechanisms that often "contaminate" our social environment, even if it is a key recommendation to not generalise individual psychodynamics to those of small and, especially, large groups, such as a population (Volkan, 2014) without a proper and deep historical context.

The International Psychoanalytical Association has encouraged the extension of psychoanalysis to reach our community, and even if many psychoanalysts have always worked in hospitals, courthouses, refugees'

DOI: 10.4324/9781003203223-19

shelters, and schools, with different types of intervention from a classical psychoanalytical setting, for a long time, the community has kept an image of the psychoanalyst as locked in his or her clinic and uninvolved in social issues, as the IPA Image Task Force has reported (Mauss-Hanke, 2015).

The United Nations was created in 1945 to prevent another world war, and since 1998, the IPA has a special consultative status in the UN, through its Economic and Social Council (ECOSOC[1]) as a non-governmental organisation. This recognition opened important meeting places to reach many people who otherwise would not benefit from psychoanalysts' help and expertise and to advocate about the psychoanalytical approach.

The IPA at the UN Subcommittee which works under the umbrella of the Humanitarian Organizations committee, has these specific tasks:

- Advocating psychoanalysis in the UN system – making IPA and psychoanalysis visible, heard, and helpful to larger section of individuals and society.
- Promoting human rights, social awareness, and international issues in the psychoanalytic community – such as conflict prevention and resolution; effects of prejudice, violence, and discrimination; and concerns about the environment, pandemics, migrations and wars, and international welfare in general.
- Creating links with other non-governmental organisations and institutions that share its commitment to mental health and psychological well-being.

Attending the UN meetings, a psychoanalyst may draw attention to the psychological suffering or traumas of individuals and populations involved in wars, migrations, violence, and abuses, often enlightening the complexity of the situations and discussing solutions, staying alert to the risk of splitting into "bad" and "good" ones in the identification of victims and perpetrators. He or she may try to clarify group dynamics correlated to socio-political situations and help gather local and international resources – for instance, creating links among other NGOs and local psychoanalytic institutes. Furthermore, in a bidirectional way, the subcommittee for the United Nations reports periodically to the IPA and its members about international issues and concerns to the psychoanalytic profession, as this chapter aims to do.

Psychoanalysis at UN meetings: a fruitful exchange

A big challenge for society today is answering with competence, appropriate tools, and human compassion to the phenomenon of migration. With COVID-19, millions of refugees lost work, and in some African states the price of the food rose by 15%; at the end of 2020, because of persecution, conflict, violence, human rights violations, and events seriously disturbing public order, 82.4 million people worldwide were forcibly displaced (to understand the huge increase, we can compare it to 2010 data, which reported about 40 million people displaced worldwide).[2]

Attending meetings and side events organised by the United Nations gives a great opportunity to interact with other NGOs (non-governmental organisations) and governmental institutions. Instead of material and concrete supplies, the IPA sets as its priority the observation and assessment of interpersonal dynamics from a psychoanalytical point of view and can offer useful perspectives. Confronting on clinical and social issues, the IPA Subcommittee for the UN informs about the work of IPA members in the community and creates links among NGO representatives, psychoanalysts, or local psychoanalytic societies.

For instance, many psychoanalysts work with migrants in individual or group consultation or supervise health care professionals and teams. Their contributions are precious for the community, and the following are only a few examples that testify the importance of sharing a specific psychoanalytic expertise in the field of migration.

Psychoanalytic crisis interventions for traumatised refugees proved to be helpful and often requires a modified psychoanalytical treatment technique (Leuzinger-Bohleber et al., 2016) but also peculiar internal settings because of the deep psychological suffering:

> [T]he migrant is in a very regressive position, a narcissistic wound because of loss of identity, job, status and because of having to rely on an NGO for food and survival and this will reenact unconsciously the traumas of the infant dependent on mother for food and shelter.
>
> (De Coster, 2017)

Health care professionals and volunteers may be unaware of this psychological point of view, of its great importance for the migrant's acceptance of the help given.

Migrants and refugees, especially if victims of tortures and rapes "sank into deep depression or psychosis with acute paranoia" (De Coster, 2017); indeed, their ability to symbolise often falls, along with their mother tongue (Kristeva, 1988; De Coster, 2017), and the communication is replaced by somatic and psychosomatic illness (De Micco, 2017; De Coster, 2017). Their main psychological mechanisms of defence are dissociation (Ferruta, 2016), denial (Egidi Morpurgo, 2016), and identification with the aggressor, which causes the reproduction of violence (Correia e Silva, 2016).

On the psychotherapist's side, a story of personal or familiar migration can bring to the enactment of mutual dissociation of their collective and personal trauma (Belkin, 2017); we can imagine that for health care professionals who have not been sustained by psychoanalytic treatment, the risk is much higher. The trauma, with its feelings of anxiety and bewilderment, may contaminate anyone who approach it, and, not unusually, it reaches even the organizations and the institutions (as described in the concept of *isomorphy* by Rene Kaës, 1976) so that they are blocked in administrative and technical difficulties (such as in the freezing reaction of the trauma) or may surrender "to the impulse to look away, to deny and to turn a blind eye to the unbearable" (Leuzinger-Bohleber et al., 2016).

In a therapeutic setting, a psychoanalyst would work with his patients to discover and understand the defence mechanisms that alter the perception of the internal and external worlds, often overcoming the dissociated and isolated part of self through a process of integration (Bromberg, 2001, 2003). In communities, integration is promoted and encouraged among migrants and the host population by NGOs and governmental institutions, but unfortunately, often, they do not examine the deep psychological reasons for racism and prejudice, linked with the history of that population and its process of "depositing" (Volkan, 2014). Also, the study of the development of large-group identities and the primitive mechanism involved are points of great interest that often open a collaboration between governments and expert psychoanalysts as consultants.

In advocating psychoanalysis to a wide variety of audiences such as in the United Nations, I have found particularly valuable the concept of "freedom." I consider it strongly connected to psychoanalysis, because patient and psychoanalyst work together not only to modify the patient's life or to eliminate symptoms, as in other kinds of psychotherapies, but to expand his/her freedom, in work, love, and life in general. Freedom is a concept that can be easily declined from the intrapsychic to interpersonal experience and is also a fundamental human right as reported in the Universal Declaration of Human Rights in 1948. In some UN meetings I introduced the International Psychoanalytical Association as an association of experts in mental health involved in the cure of the victims, in the training of the health professionals, and in initiatives that promote mental health and the value of intrapsychic and interpersonal freedom.

My first experience was at the seventh session of the Conference of the Parties to the UN Convention against Transnational Organized Crime, held in Vienna from 6 to 10 October 2014. The side events organised by the NGOs were the appropriate places to raise attention on mental health issues and on the IPA and to confront about projects against human trafficking and the empowerment of women and harmful traditional practices, such as female genital mutilation.

People were interested in the psychoanalytical approach which has its roots in clinical experience but also includes psychosocial issues. For example, we discussed the relationship between domestic violence and human trafficking in Albany, where beaten wives, who find the courage to divorce, are no longer supported by their families and have a greater risk of being caught in sex trafficking. In this situation some measures were proposed, such as psychological support to the victims of violence and psychoanalytic supervision to the group of operators that work for them – often all women as well, fighting a patriarchal culture.

The importance of awareness of the population through public debate and the education of new generations for a more profound and persistent "change of mind"was also discussed. With Maria Falcone, sister of the judge Giovanni Falcone, killed by the mafia in 1992, we deepened the subject of education about legality in schools, the lack of paternal function in modern society, and the importance of international cooperation and a shared understanding of the "human" nature of crime and antisocial tendencies, following Winnicott's theory of deprivation (1956, 2011).

During the yearly Geneva Peace Week (GPW),[3] at the panel titled "Women's meaningful participation in peacemaking: lessons from global leaders," the speakers, sitting at a huge, square table with all of us participants, affirmed that what makes the difference for reaching and implementing sustainable peace agreements is the level of influence that women have on the process – not merely their numerical presence ("making women count, not just counting women"). Statistical research reported that whenever women's groups have been able to participate and influence negotiations or push for a peace deal since its very beginning (in pre-negotiation), an agreement has almost always been reached, while when women's groups are not involved at all, or have only minimal influence on the process, the chance of reaching an agreement is considerably lower. Psychoanalysis can further reflect that overcoming divisions and building coalitions are not abilities directly and exclusively referred to women but represents a feminine function that can no longer be synonymous of passivity nor merely containment, but also reflects the perseverance and the ability to maintain relationships, as explored in depth in our recent IPA Congress in London, in 2019.

Other interactive panels at the GPW discussed new policy developments, research, and case studies about non-violent action, peacebuilding, and interfaith dialogue, as tools for conflict prevention and resolution. A psychoanalyst can fully understand the assertion that "conflicts sometimes are necessary" and that a shift from "conflict prevention" to "violence prevention" may sometimes, or for a certain time, also be necessary.

Since 2020, the Geneva Peace Week has taken place online and emphasised that the global pandemic has been widening inequalities and racial conflicts at an unprecedented scale, with a big concern about the reduction of global solidarity, due to the focus on survival efforts, local solidarity, and nationalism. Speaking of disparities, I observed huge differences among the places where the several panelists connected from: some of them video-called from nice rooms with libraries and paintings, others from courtyards, poor buildings, or noisy offices, and others had to drive many miles to reach a town where they could have internet connection. Recently, psychological issues gained more attention, and the mechanism of denial of the virus in the population was largely recognised and discussed. Another theme regarded the identity process from former combatants to become and remain local "peacebuilders,"[4] where a social worker recognised in a former combatant the Freudian slip between the words "coffee" and "conflict" – that facilitated the revelation of her diffidence and then the development of a more genuine group discussion. At the panel on social media and democracy, instead of talking about the increase of hate speech and hate crimes in Europe, the debate was blocked at the question "if hate comes from fear, where fear comes from?" And I believe that psychoanalysts should engage in searching for an answer.

Local projects and world community

Another way to advocate psychoanalysis is promoting contributions about areas of international concern, through participation in local community projects. As stated by Filippo Grandi, UN High Commissioner for Refugees, in his video celebration of the 2019 World Refugee Day:

> [R]efugees themselves need to be included in new communities and given the chance to realize their potential. . . . Getting laws and policies right is vital. But it is local people and communities that are on the frontlines when refugees arrive, and whose welcome makes the difference – the difference between rejection and inclusion; between despair and hope; between being left behind and building a future. Sharing responsibility for refugees starts there.

The arrival in the host country is often problematic, at high risk of solicitation into slavery or prostitution. The migrants feel disoriented and often experience conflictual emotions towards their relatives because it is difficult to accept what they ask them to do to save the rest of the family (De Micco, 2017). Host countries do not seem prepared to face the challenge of migration and recognise its potentiality, and psychoanalysis observes that their population usually becomes polarised in its social response (Volkan, 2014), including the web and social media (Vermote, 2017) that are showing to be exceptionally important in influencing the population and should be carefully studied from a psychoanalytical point of view.

The crisis of meta-psychic and meta-social guarantors described by Kaës (2007) has created a situation in which dislocated subjects (the natives) host other dislocated subjects (the migrants) (De Micco, 2017), ending in episodes of intolerance and violence, and this brought many psychoanalysts to decide to leave their chairs behind their couches, for a while, and participate in social activities to help local communities and the world community.

In the project "Adolescents and Migrants: Poetry of Resistance and Play,"[5] carried out in Rimini, Italy, for three years, the targets were students from high schools and young refugees. Since the formation of a solid individual identity finalises during adolescence along with large-group identity, and endures throughout a lifetime (Volkan, 2014), it is very important to reach and sustain psychologically this passage of life, also as a form of protection of the population's future mental health and because it is at higher risk of religious radicalisation and fundamentalism (Bennani, 2018; Hirsch, 2018).

The common theme of the journey was creatively elaborated through many artistic forms (drawing, poetry, drama and music workshops, short films) with the help of artists and musicians. The journey had a concrete meaning for migrants and refugees, while students recalled the passage to adult life. Students and migrants, coordinated by a psychoanalyst, shared their experiences and thoughts about violence, human's right violations, bullying, and prejudice and examined in depth the themes of diversity and multiplicity in gender, culture, and religion. The project had a strong impact on the community through the final public show and the video, which promoted awareness to the themes of migrants and refugees and the tolerance of diversity and helped to overcome isolation during the COVID-19 lockdown.

I also got pleasantly involved in "The Tail of the Game," a photographic project by Matteo Placucci, who travelled in Bosnia and Herzegovina in January 2021 to meet migrants approaching the Balkan Route to the European Union. He focused on single men between 15 and 40 years old, the majority in numbers but perceived as the less vulnerable category (compared to women and children) and consequently with fewer possibilities to be admitted into the receptive structures, such as the temporary reception centres (TRC) for asylum seekers near the Croatian border. They miss physical and psychological support and often find compensation in alcohol and drug abuse, started as self-medication, while waiting for the winter season to finish and try the "game" – that is, the final passage to the EU through a trip that takes from two to three weeks between crossing Croatia and Slovenia and reaching Italy.

> *Roohullah, 19 years old, from Afghanistan, uses alcohol to ease his kidney pain. He is a poet, and whenever he feels bad, he brings back the poetry from his mind "to give me strength." In his dream he sees himself working in Italy, wants to learn the native language and apply for an education: "Europe needs talented and good educated people."*

Most migrants try the game several times, sometimes dozens of times, but often, they are forced back to Bosnia and Herzegovina, after being beaten by the police and having all their belongings stolen. This situation is legitimated by governments that deny their rights as asylum seekers and by the indifference of the community.

> *Shabaz is 25 and comes from Afghanistan in an extremely poor family. He lost his father three months ago and was advised by his brother in a phone call in the very middle of his ninth Game, making him unable to go forward. The hardest threats to his psychological stability are still the phone calls from his brothers, asking him why he is unable to pass the border. He has mostly bad dreams: "I was in a car and was going around in a circle, waiting for the impact of a crash." He recalls a serious car crash in the mountains, when they were illegally entering Greece from Turkey, but also connects it to his stuck situation.*
>
> *The life of Rizwan, 20 years old, from Pakistan, is marked by the trauma of trying the Game with a family in Bihać, "they were traveling with babies, but unable to carry them, and the babies fell down the mountains." He does not link, however, this episode to his abuse of drugs and alcohol.*

The photographer in his interviews of the migrants focused on their mental status and asked for a psychoanalyst's help to develop a questionnaire that could help in investigating their stories and getting in touch with their feelings, without hurting them. The questionnaire consists of 25 questions and asks about family and some crucial moments of the present and ends on their desire for the future. It alternates specific questions, such as anamnestic data and quality of sleep, with more open ones, to facilitate free associations, such as "what is the first thing that comes up when you think about your home country?" Other questions confront them with emotional conflict: "how do you feel when you think about your family?" and "have you ever thought about going back?" We thought that this could give a chance for emotions and feelings to emerge, or be easily avoided and denied, in a similar way to a projective test. Reading some of the interviews, several symptoms of severe depression and PTSD emerged, such as traumas, flashbacks, and nightmares, but also the importance of dreams in their life: to stay connected to their family and their lost countries, to remember their mission and destination, and to encourage their journey, giving them the opportunity to elaborate psychological trauma in images instead of words. Policemen often populate the nightmares of several migrants, seeding a higher risk for an upheaval between justice and illegality that often confirms the corrupted system experienced in their country of origin, causing a deep painful disenchantment. But since they carry the burden to save the family from war or release it from poverty, for the great part of them, this is a one-way street, and the violence of the pushbacks does not affect their mission.

> *Farid is 31 and emigrated for economic reasons: "in Morocco even if you are working, the money is not enough to survive. It is like riding a bicycle and*

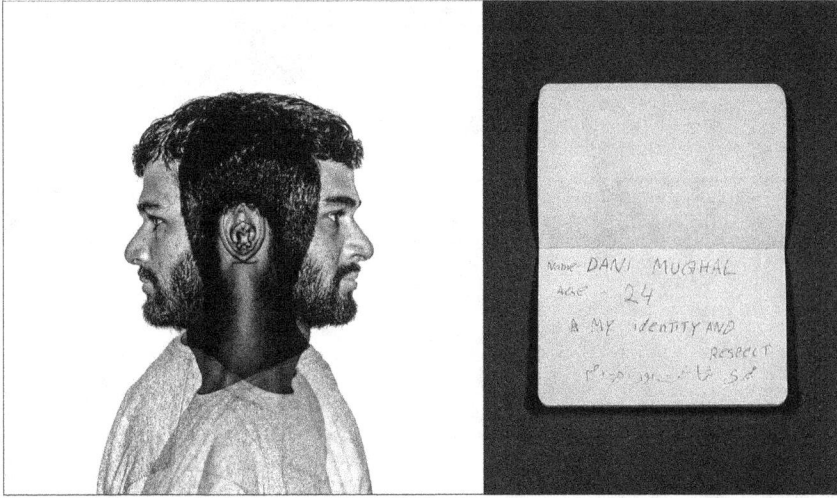

Figure 16.1 Matteo Placucci Photography, project "The Tail of the Game-Balkan Route."

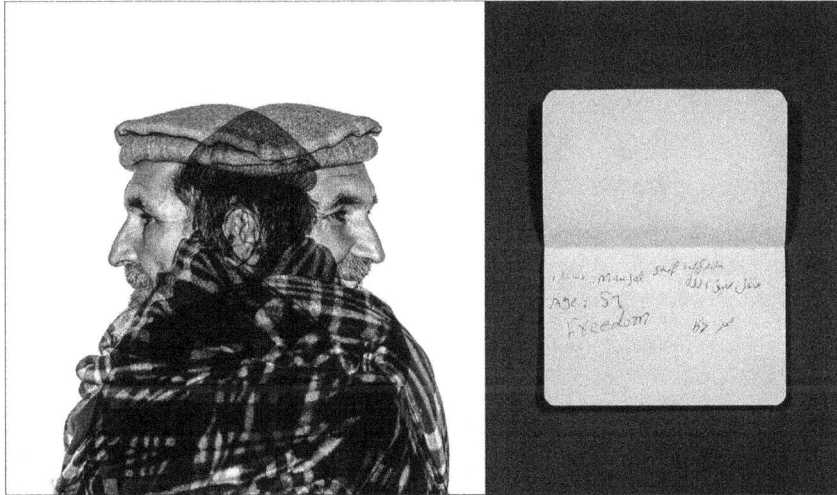

Figure 16.2 Matteo Placucci Photography, project "The Tail of the Game-Balkan Route."

going nowhere, being stuck always in the same place." He regrets having left, especially after a truck crash that causes the loss of his right leg and phantom pain. "That day I thought about going back to my mom in Morocco, but suddenly I realized that for being handicapped, my mother could not provide for me." He continues to experience the trauma through his dream: "when I saw

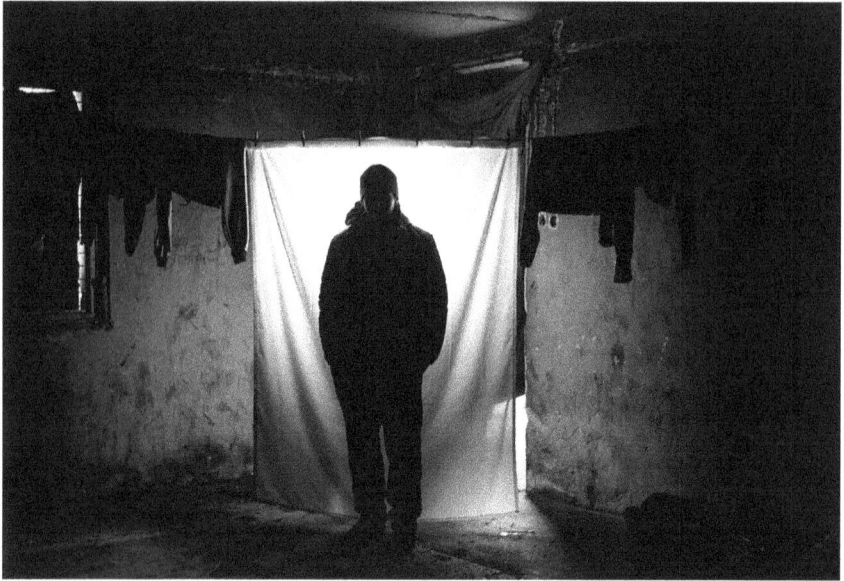

Figure 16.3 Matteo Placucci Photography, project "The Tail of the Game-Balkan Route."

the truck that hit me and lost my leg. But the story in the dream is different: it is a gang from the local mafia that drives the truck, or that wants to cut my leg."

Matteo Placucci's pictures capture their double look: to the past and to the future, creating a sort of modern representation of the Rorschach tables, where the migrants are themselves the inkblots of the tables.

Conclusions

Wars, environmental disasters, and inequalities in economic resources are some causes of migration and require a collective answer from experts in mental health. Psychoanalysts are trained to work with psychological trauma and to *hold* and *handle* (Winnicott, 1958) affective wounds and primitive defences that occur in refugees, migrants, and in host populations, which the COVID-19 pandemic has been widening. Psychoanalysis proved to be helpful not only as a psychotherapy for the victims, but also in the prevention of trauma and burnout of the health professionals and helping a deeper understanding of individual and group dynamics. At a social level, psychoanalysis may help to promote processes of integration

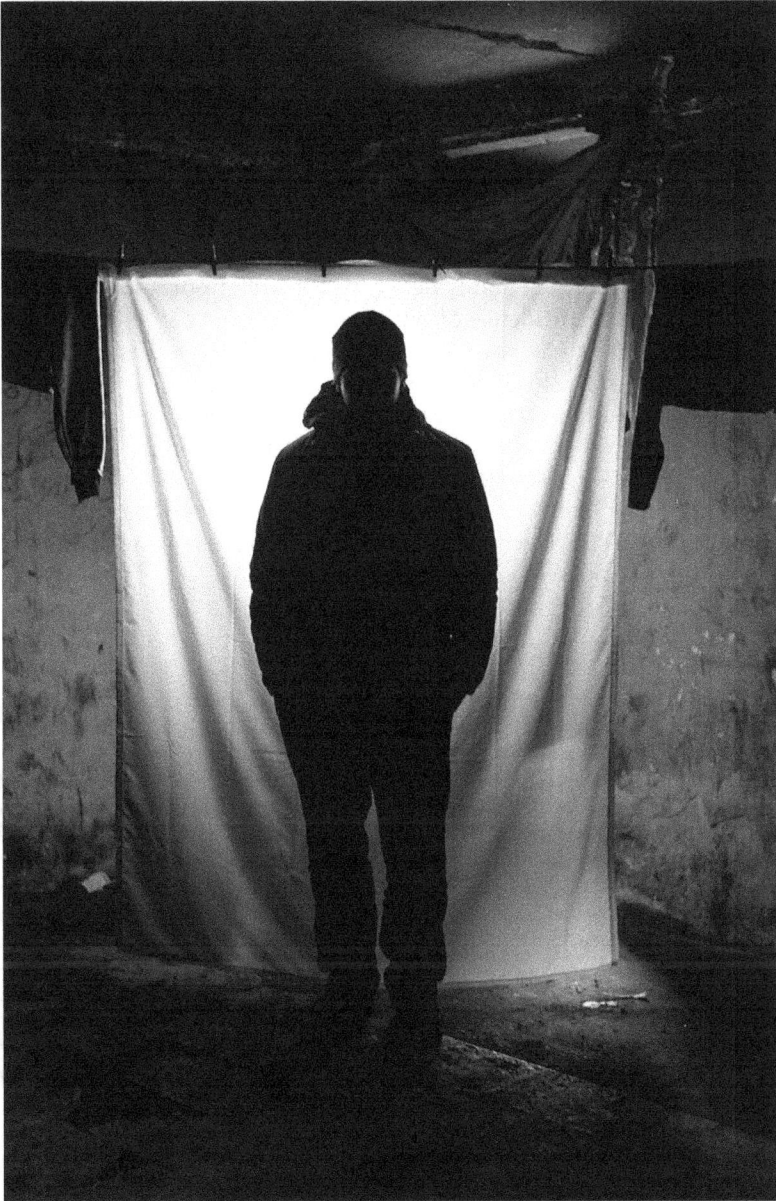

Figure 16.4 Matteo Placucci Photography, project "The Tail of the Game-Balkan Route."

and the value of intrapsychic and interpersonal freedom especially in the young population, often by means of arts, in each form (music, painting, sculpture, cinema, or photography) and the United Nations system is an important place to reach people and organisations and to share psycho-analysts' expertise.

In conclusion, I think it is useful to remember that the UN has been highly criticised for not having carried out its mission to maintain inter-national peace and security or solving international problems, because it permits us a last reflection. The debates about it are considered often aca-demic and radicalised (Bertrand, 1995) and, as previously said, a psycho-analyst should be alerted by language that opposes *us* to *others* and that cancels any possibility of ambivalence, but, more important, I believe this is part of a general diffidence of our society towards any institution, and that a similar feeling affects us and the IPA as well, felt as distant from our clinical practice or the local psychoanalytic institutes.

It may be explained as a basic assumption of dependency (Bion, 1961) that delegates to others our responsibility and that is linked to our own – as human beings – resistance to change.

Recalling Patti Smith's song, I wish our profession to *have the power* to use – and share – our psychoanalytic tools to overcome some of this resist-ance and involve ourselves in the community.

Notes

1 ECOSOC is one of the six major organs of the United Nations, its heart and main platform of debate and proposal to set international common goals.
2 See for updates: www.unhcr.org/flagship-reports/globaltrends/
3 Geneva Peace Week is a collective action initiative facilitated by the United Nations Office at Geneva (UNOG), the Graduate Institute for International and Development Studies, and the Geneva Peacebuilding Platform in collaboration with the Swiss Confederation. By synchronising meetings on different topics related to the promotion of peace, this one-week event underlines that each per-son, actor, and institution has a role to play in building peace and resolving conflict and that peace promotion occurs in many different contexts, disciplines, and sectors.
4 Organised by the Gender Centre, Muhammadiyah University of Madiun, and the Swiss Program for Research on Global Issues for Development.
5 "Adolescents and migrants: poetry of resistance and play" is a project coordi-nated by Cinzia Carnevali, Laura Ravaioli, and Gabriella Vandi and the winner of the 2021 IPA in the Community Award for the Section IPA in Education.

References

Belkin M. (2017). Carrying the burden of loss across the ocean: Transmission of trauma in migrant families. *Psychoanalysis Today*, Issue 3, Migration.
Bertrand, M. (1995). The UN as an organization. A critique of its Functioning. *Euro-pean Journal of International Law*, 6(3), 349–359.

Bennani, J. (2018, febbraio 3). L'adolescente alla prova dell'esilio. In *Giornata di studio internazionale Menti Migranti, Menti adolescenti Tra sradicamenti e radicalizzazioni*. Paper at the Congress in Firenze.

Bion, W. R. (1961). *Experiences in groups*. London: Tavistock.

Bromberg P. M. (2001). Out of body, out of mind, out of danger. In J. Petrucelli & C. Stuart (Eds.), *Hungers and compulsions*. Northvale, NJ: Aronson.

Bromberg, P. M. (2003). One need not be a house to be haunted: On enactment, dissociation, and the dread of "Not-Me" – A case study. *Psychoanalytic Dialogues, 13*, 689–709.

Correia e Silva Filinto Elísio. (2016). Some contributions to understanding violence in (and of) the Cape Verdean community in Portugal. *Psychoanalysis Today*, Issue 2, Violence.

Davids, M. F. (2011). *Internal racism. A Psychoanalytic approach to race and difference*. London: Red Globe Press.

De Coster, N. (2017). The other language: A few psychoanalytic thoughts about migration, the loss of culture and language. *Psychoanalysis Today*, Issue 3, Migration.

De Micco, V. (2017). Migrare. Sopravvivere al disumano. *Rivista italiana di Psicoanalisi* (4).

Egidi Morpurgo, V. (2016). Harbouring pain. A clinical undertaking and an ethical duty. *Forum on Collective Traumas*. Paper at the Congress of the European Psychoanalytical Federation, Berlin.

Ferruta, A. (2016). Psychoanalysis as a discipline of the living beings. What we can learn from the effective tragedies of contemporaneity: the tragedies of drowned immigrants. *Forum on Collective Traumas*. Paper at the Congress of the European Psychoanalytical Federation, Berlin.

Hirsch, D. (2018). La presa in ostaggio del sé adolescente nella radicalizzazione religiosa: identificazione alienante, sradicamento, identitario, melancolizzazione nella cultura. In *Giornata di studio internazionale Menti Migranti, Menti adolescenti Tra sradicamenti e radicalizzazioni*. Paper at the Congress in Firenze.

Kaës, R. (1976). *L'appareil psychique groupal*. Paris: Dunod.

Kaës, R. (2007). *Linking, alliances, and shared space, groups and the psychoanalyst*. London: Routledge.

Kristeva, J. (1988). *Strangers to ourselves*. New York: Columbia University Press, 1991.

Leuzinger-Bohleber, M., Rickmeyer, C., Tahiri, M., Hettic, N., & Fischmann, T. (2016). What can psychoanalysis contribute to the current refugee crisis. *International Journal of Psychoanalysis, 97*(4), 1077–1093.

Mauss-Hanke, A. (2015, July). *Images of psychoanalysis- The work of the IPA image task force*. Panel at the IPA Congress, Boston.

Vermote, R. (2017). Refugees: A confusion of tongues. *Psychoanalysis Today*, Issue 3, Migration.

Volkan, V. D (2014). *Psychoanalysis, international relations and diplomacy*. London: Karnac Book.

Winnicott, D. W. (1958). *Collected papers. Through paediatrics to psycho-analysis*. London: Tavistock Publications.

Winnicott, D. W. (1956). *The antisocial tendency in "deprivation and delinquency"*. London: Routledge, 2011.

17 The psychoanalyst, psychoanalysis, and human rights

A perspective that instigates us

Paola Amendoeira

Introduction

> *A turkey, in the center of a circle outlined by chalk, is said to feel irreparably a prisoner of the circle. One day, I thought I should escape to freedom, jumping out of the circle. I cut the ties that held me down to all social conventions and to this gentle comfort of repeated habits. I moved forward. Now brooding over recent experiences, comparing them to old ones, I realize that life is nothing but a succession of concentric chalk circles. We jump out of one just to find out that we are prisoners of another, and then another. It is the human condition.*
>
> (Veríssimo, 2006)

Henceforth, in face of this unsettling and endless saga, I head for this endless psychoanalytic future.

We will have to face so many changes, so many deconstructions, and so many disillusionments. Becoming a psychoanalyst is personal and irreplaceable, but it is an experience that needs meeting points, exchanges, support, acceptance, and above all, bonds of belonging.

It is possible, however undesirable, to go through this saga (this experience) unharmed.

It is painful to decide to jump out of the circle just to find another circle, and another, and many others. Moreover, in this way, we start broadening our horizons, rethinking our goals, reevaluating our dreams, and perhaps then, we can learn to enjoy this bizarre and unique journey. In recognising our limitations, we can tolerate our frustrations and contribute to the society we live in.

> In Freud's, psychoanalysis took up a much larger area than just the consulting room therapy; after him, inside the psychoanalytic movement, psychoanalysis did not evolve; it shrank, though. The psychoanalytic theory, easily adapted to the practice, turning into individual psychology and the psychoanalyst training split up into scholastic doctrinal systems. The same political agreements that determine the psychoanalytic power centers have established the permissible

DOI: 10.4324/9781003203223-20

extension of the clinic and, by association, the level of theorization, thus defining the standard clinic and the standard theory.

(Hermann, 2003, p. 168)

It is worth mentioning that in his work on group psychology and ego analysis, Freud stated that individual psychology is also social psychology, and he emphasised the interconnections among individuals and their cultures (Penna, 2014).

Nowadays, we can see how societies, their institutes, and psychoanalysts themselves revisit the Freudian texts held as social. Books like *Uneasiness in Culture, The Future of an Illusion, The Ego and Mass Psychology, Totem and Taboo,* and *Moses and Monotheism* present a possible and sensitive reflection of the vicissitudes of the death drive, astonishment, and prejudice and violence deriving from them.

In Brazil, for example, the Psychoanalytic Observatory was created in 2017. It is a forum where psychoanalysts expose their ideas about varied subjects, sociopolitical, cultural, or institutional, under a psychoanalytic vertex. The PO, as it is informally called, holds a space like a revenant virtual agora, in which psychoanalysts are invited to reflect on the subject of the unconscious and its relation with the world and the present time they live in.

In national or international congresses, we see a couch that moves around.[1] Since the beginning of the century, working accounts began to appear and stimulate the psychoanalyst's experience in a broader setting. More and more reflection and acceptance groups were formed to deal with the suffering of those who live in recurrent traumatic situations, which erode the capacity of psychic work because of the violence and social vulnerability they experience.

The psychoanalyst finds himself in a situation of disquieting astonishment. He is sometimes invited, sometimes internally or extraneously summoned, to help in the construction of a space where wild thoughts in their origin may be primarily analysed, and perhaps find some type of destination. Is it domestication or permanence in the category of discomfort?

When mentioning the extensive clinic, Hermann reminds us how deeply psychoanalysis (beyond the standard clinic) has established itself as the science of man.

The International Psychoanalytic Association (IPA), attentive to its roots, created a table of values for its members. IPA ethical principles reflect humanitarian values and have in their constitution items referring to human rights, such as "No psychoanalyst will take part in or will stimulate the violation of human rights basic to any individual, as is defined by the Declaration of the Human Rights in the UN."

Based on ideas of freedom, equality, and fraternity among men, the Declaration of Human Rights was adopted by the United Nations in 1948 and last year celebrated its 73rd year of existence.

We certainly expected to be face to face with an elderly woman, full of experience, maturity, a rich memory, and history. However, what we are met with is volatility, liquidity, and ephemerality. It is another time. Not the chronological time of a human life, though. It is a slower, denser, complex time that moves quickly to stagnation. How long did it take men to discover and control fire? From fire to cooking? From cooking to a house? From a house to the fireplace? From the fireplace to the idea of a family? From family to the invention of childhood? From the invention of the wheel to the trip to the moon?

The wheel of time keeps spinning faster and faster with globalisation, information technology, and the net, with less permanence and more, a lot more, ephemerality.

Bauman (1997/1998) believes that postmodernity is ruled by the failure of the universal metanarratives that today seem to be old, anachronistic, and fading constellations. Things that were shared before, lose their leading roles to the supremacy of the so-called "I think that . . . "

It looks as if the search for truth, equality, and fraternity is not a goal anymore but a constraint, which must be socially denied, suppressed, and abolished.

Reality strongly knocks on our door to remind us that human rights are not a finishing line, ready, and completed, but a continuous, persistent, and permanent movement.

Utopia (?)

Human Rights are remembered when they are violated or ravished.
(Viñar, 2008)

Psychoanalysis and history

When Freud created and developed psychoanalysis, there came about a possibility, a capacity of an open space, an open mind to explain what was apparently considered absurd. Why listen to mad people? Why listen to women with symptoms of conversion disorder?

Freud is contemporary of a constellation called traditional, bourgeois, nuclear, patriarchal, and monogamist family – a time when hysterical conversions expressed and denounced a violent sexual repression against sexuality as a whole, but mainly against the woman.

Thus, brilliantly, Freud revealed the unconscious universal fantasy, shared by men and women, that women are castrated beings. Harold Blum, quoted by Young-Bruehl (1996), says

"For the first time, there was a scientific understanding of the contempt and the derision toward women based upon overdetermined, irrational unconscious fantasies. Both boys and girls and their parents unconsciously regarded the female as castrated and, therefore, inferior." Viewing Freud as a liberator, Blum could conclude with a view of the "female as having diminished and constrained libido, a weaker and masochistic sexual constitution, an ego with an incapacity to sublimate and a tendency toward early arrest and rigidity, a relatively defective superego, and incomplete oedipal and preoedipal development" – that is, with a view of the female as, *in fact*, not in irrational fantasy, castrated.

(Young-Bruehl, 1996, p. 284)

The dispute over the domain of human comprehension has created, initially, a radical splitting, distancing and preventing the integration between social understanding and the psychological theories that provided an understanding of the human at an individual level. In the upbringing of these sciences still in development, they seemed to be more focused on the strengthening of their identities and in the recognising and demarcating of their territories. This split paralysed thinking, made it impossible to recognise and be aware of the place from which one speaks and of the vertex that determines its range of vision and action.

The great contribution offered by psychoanalysis is that it is a tool to call the attention and accommodate what is diverse to the system, but which is at the same time our system, a part of ourselves, a part for which our expectations were not prepared and should have remained secretive, buried, but that came to light (Freud, 1919/2019).

Psychoanalysis opens a special listening to the human suffering, and it only grows if it can only expand, if it can welcome and be attentive of the understanding that some particular circumstances are promoted by different psychosocial contexts or backgrounds that are culturally passed on through particular shared unconscious phantasies.

For more than 20 years, the IPA has been a non-governmental organisation at the UN, ascribed with special consultative status. Through its UN Subcommittee, the IPA does not stay silent in the face of human rights abuses and violations. It has its opinion heard and can be consulted regarding the mental health issues of individuals and populations. We have the task of making psychoanalysis visible and heard not only in the United Nations System but also in the meetings of the Economic and Social Council and its subsidiary bodies.

Through the IPA's Subcommittee for the UN, psychoanalysis is applied to human tragedies, which are also political if we consider the Aristotelian sense of the term.

The interface between the IPA and UN is a large two-way road. Our presence contributes to the prevention and resolution of conflicts and the discussion of the effects of racial, religious, and ethnic prejudice; gender identity; child abuse; and violence (Sayad, 2008). When our voice is heard, it is possible to raise awareness of all the international community to the importance of the little-remembered emotional impact and its psychic consequences on the mental health of those who might have their rights threatened or violated. International forums, as well as psychoanalysis itself all benefit from the opportunity to think, develop, and deepen our science, updating it and, above all, "reconnecting us with a responsibility that seems inevitable" (Marinho, 2005). We can offer our knowledge and our great raw material about the subjectivity of the human experience in favour of the common good.

And it is in this sense that the IPA has been affirming itself as an important civil society actor with great potential to promote the civic space, which is the heart of the social fabric and contract. The IPA is a beacon, a beam of light that illuminates a possible path and is precise to place racism and prejudice at the heart of the discussion.

We have vast knowledge; various tools to share; and a brilliant field that has been inviting us to penetrate, learn, and perhaps, broaden our view. The work is arduous, unlimited, and painful sometimes, but deeply urgent and necessary nowadays.

In 2014, when participating in the Conference of the Parts of the Convention of Nations against organised and transnational crime in Vienna, Laura Ravaioli spoke of the interest shown by the participants in relation to the psychoanalytic approach. It is an important experience that makes clear that we have a large space to (re)occupy, being only necessary that we go beyond the frames of our consulting rooms, so that we remain in them alive, enriched, updated, and above all, attentive.

The feminine

Alongside his studies, Freud experienced a growing restlessness. He admitted his limitation to understanding women more deeply and confessed to understanding the masculine oedipal unfolding better, which he recognised as simpler than women's evolvement. He repeatedly stated that women needed to start studying psychoanalysis and working as psychoanalysts so that a deeper understanding of their oedipal experience and of the feminine perception could be achieved. Thus, we realise Freud was an enthusiastic stimulator of women in psychoanalysis. Women's dedication to psychoanalysis has enriched this field, adding new discussions to the themes.

Today we are here at a subcommittee not only presided over by a woman but also composed by many other women in its body.

However, despite a massive feminine participation, few of the women's productions are studied. There is a prevalence of papers written by men. We ask therefore an uncomfortable question: why is that?

In spite of this massive feminine presence in institutes and societies, it took 110 years for the IPA to have its first female president. It is possible, though, to find a female chair of committees, president of societies, or directors of institutes. We have a lot to reflect and work on these themes.

> Moreover, since the world is world, discussion on the feminine enigma is crossed over by the relationship established with the masculine. From an early age, the human being has experienced rivalry with the other sex they carry inside of them.
>
> (Gerchmann, 2019)

The search for equality of gender in the family, at work, and in society as a whole and the prevention and elimination of violence against women, either middle aged, young, or children have been rapidly evolving; at the same time that some differences seem to be upsurging. Women, on the one hand, have been broadening their territory of self-experiences with their bodies and the ones around them, assuming their femininity and their accomplishment beyond marriage and maternity. Now they are recognised by the values that they foster and support.

On the other hand, we still notice a high degree of violence and ravishment of their rights to equality, which may sometimes be expressed by the opposite sex. An arrangement is established in which satisfaction is guaranteed, on the one hand, but that instigates intolerance on the other. There arises a certain difficulty in accepting, bearing, or even enjoying the encounter with the difference and with the other who thus becomes as alien as women to the opposite sex. The pendulum sways from one side to the other, but it cannot alter or go beyond the polarity that it represents.

With all the clinical experience we have accumulated, we have the capacity to help and even change the route as far as we can express the importance and pleasure that the acceptance of the difference or the relationship with the opposites will bring back in terms of pleasure, accomplishment, transformation, and creativity.

We have to create spaces for the elaboration of this hatred, cultivated by both poles, almost ontogenetically built, so that it will not have to be operated and may find new and more creative destinations.

Migrants

> History shows that omission is not innocent and the closing one's eyes, lying and shutting silent also make perish . . . humanity.
>
> (Gerchmann, 2019)

We have been concerned with the various branches of the UN system for the refugees. The UNHCR is the UN agency for the refugees and it aids in the management of the forced displacement of people in a global scale and mitigation of violations of human rights.

In the clinical work, psychoanalysts often demand the presence of an interpreter. However, social workers or supervised medical assistance could help indirectly. It is a practice that broadens the range of psychoanalysis and requires not only a technique of a modified psychoanalytic treatment (Leuzinger-Bohleber, 2016), (Hermann, 2003), but also creates a peculiar internal setting due to its deep psychological suffering.

The experience of migration, naturally traumatic, activates anxieties and primitive defences associated with strong feelings of helplessness, bringing up a special sensitivity to the experience of corporal separation between self and the object. Several accounts of insomnia, maladaptation to new customs, avoidance of personal contact, strong memories of the family and the life left behind abound. The migrant experiences feelings of distrust, which make them isolated (Rosa & Nogueira, 2017). On the other hand, when they overcome this resistance to contact, they may develop a more "adhesive" relationship.

When one is forced to migrate, for social, political, economic, or individual motivations, he feels exposed to a variety of situations of social vulnerability, among which is the risk of subjective or real slavery encouraged by a strong need of belonging.

Conclusion

In this scenario, psychoanalysis contributes to a special listening that constantly calls us to the exercise of what Bion alluded as without memory and without desire. The exercise of a kind of self-attention to implicit and unconscious prejudices and the fantasies that engender them is the discipline that enables us to embrace the sufferings arising from the migrant experience in search of finding their place in a new society, respecting the subjective singularities in transit and helplessness.

> The signature of an Anthropological Psychoanalysis is another idea that supports such experiences, as Herrmann describes in an unprecedented comment, in 2006: "The task of expanding the clinic imposes consideration to the problem of psychoanalytic listening taking place outside the culture where Psychoanalysis was born. An anthropology of psychoanalytic knowledge. It shows that psychoanalytic listening is listening psychoanalytically to what is already there. It is not inventing psychoanalysis from a certain place but learning from the place without forcing the senses."
>
> (Khouri, 2017)

The fundamental approach for the present human being is to have eyes that hear, accept, and search for rescue for a connection (belonging) and a deserved existence and fight for the rights of the minorities, political prisoners, and exiles. Moreover, to end up, I would like to say that this work is important to that population, but it is as important and pertinent to those who can exert and be committed to ethics and human existence. Let us grow in number!

Note

1 Referring to Fabio Herrmann's *Divã à Passeio (The moving couch)*.

References

Bauman, Z. (1998). *O Mal estar da pós-modernidade* (M. Gama & C. M. Gama, Trans.). Brazil, Rio de Janeiro: Zahar (Original work published in 1997).

Freud, S. (2019). *O infamiliar* (E. Chaves & P. H. Tavares, Trans.). Brazil, Belo Horizonte: Autêntica Editora (Original work published in 1919).

Gerchmann, A. (2019). *Guerra em tempos de paz*. Unpublished work.

Hermann, F. (2003). A Travessia da Incerteza. *Jornal de Psicanálise – O Homem e a Adversidade: Investigação, Teoria e Clínica Psicanalíticas*, 36(66–67), 167–194.

Khouri, M. (2017). *Por que não Psicanálise? A Clínica psicanalítica acessível na relação com a cidade*. Unpublished work presented at the Psychoanalytic Observatory of SBPSP.

Leuzinger-Bohleber, M., Rickmeyer, C., Tahiri, M., Hettich, N., & Fischmann, T. (2016). What can psychoanalysis contribute to the current refugee crisis? Preliminary reports from STEP-BY-STEP: A psychoanalytic pilot project for supporting refugees in a "first reception camp" and crisis interventions with traumatized refugees. *The International Journal of Psychoanalysis*, 97(4), 1077–1093. https://doi.org/10.1111/1745-8315.12542

Marinho, N. (2005). *Barbárie, terrorismo e psicanálise*. Retrieved from https://psicod.org/barbrie-terrorismo-e-psicanlise.html

Penna, C. (2014). *Inconsciente social*. Brazil, São Paulo: Casa do Psicólogo/Pearson.

Rosa, M. D., & Nogueira, T. S. (2017). Intimidade e Alteridade: A experiência do refúgio e a clínica psicanalítica. *Calibán, Revista Latinoamericana de Psicoanálisis*, 15(1).

Sayad, M. (2008). *Objetivo, Função e Participação do Comitê da IPA (IPACUN) na ONU – Out.2006 – e no Congresso de Berlim – Jul. 2007*. Unpublished work presented at the first Scientific Meeting of the Brazilian Society of Psychoanalysis at Rio de Janeiro.

Veríssimo, E. (2006). *Saga*. Brazil, São Paulo: Companhia das Letras.

Viñar, M. (2008). Derechos Humanos y Psicoanálisis. *Calibán, Revista Latinoamericana de Psicoanálisis*, 8.

Young-Bruehl, E. (1996). *The anatomy of prejudices*. Cambridge, MA: Harvard University Press.

18 The right to stay in place

Sargam Jain

In a book about migration, it occurred to me that we should examine the companion of movement, which is *to stay*. Correspondingly, if we are considering migration as a phenomenon that has psychic repercussions such as trauma, then staying in place necessarily also has its own mental construct and effects.

To stay somewhere is an essential activity of human beings. We exist in dimensions of time and space. Perhaps, in a quantum sense, we are constantly moving through both, but the lived reality of human experience is that it always occurs in a spatial, earthbound environment that is more or less constant over some period of time. For the purposes of clarity and brevity, let us refer to the combination of human activity within a space on the earth, as "place" (Malpas, 1998, p. 36). "Place," in this chapter, refers to a particular quality of human existence itself, not to a location or a physical extension to which feelings attach themselves or as a purely subjective experience of one's surroundings. Placed-ness is a mode of being that is always present and what is disrupted in migratory processes. A stable placed-ness, which could be characterised as feeling at home in the world, is vital to a sense of self and as such should be considered a constitutive element of a person's humanity. The formation of a stable situated self, of placed-ness, I argue, requires a continuity of physical environment which is at first coextensive with one's mother.[1] Over time, this maternal-environmental matrix of infancy is internalised and self-managed. That is all to say: *there is a human psychological requirement for a stable and personally organised geography for a healthy life.*

This geographical requirement is easily overlooked in areas of study and policy pertaining to the meaning of being human because it is so fundamental. This oversight has significant consequences, particularly for the consideration of human rights. The Universal Declaration of Human Rights ratified by the United Nations in 1948 represents the broadest global consensus on the basic existential requirements for a human life. Initially signed by 58 countries, it now counts 148 total signatories (Samnøy, 1993). A global anxiety about the murderous drives unleashed during a decade

DOI: 10.4324/9781003203223-21

of war found expression and relief in this new set of commandments, a communal psychic protection against the "brute force" of the individual (Freud, 1961a, p. 95). The declaration is a guarantee of humanity. It is also a prohibition against dehumanisation and the sadism this tendency both requires and provokes.

If the right to stay in a place were an article of the declaration, then the involuntary displacement of people through the destruction of their places of living would be considered, at the very least, a cause for sanction. It would certainly be a dehumanising act. But this is not the case – it occurs now, daily, all over the world: in the exercise of eminent domain in American cities,[2] in the destruction of ancestral Uighur villages by the Chinese government (Maizland, 2021),[3] and in the drowned towns flooded by development projects like the Mandal or Ilisu Dam (Gall, 2020).[4] It is not hard to imagine that it hurts a person to have their home bulldozed, neighbours scattered, and familiar architecture torn down. In a phenomenon she calls "root shock," Mindy Fullilove documents the traumatic stress that results for people and communities when neighbourhoods are destroyed (Fullilove, 2005).

Yet, the right to stay in place is not in the declaration. What is? The articles can be broadly separated into two categories: descriptions of *human characteristics* and the *modes of being human*. The former are described within the declaration as:

- the capacity for reason (Article I)
- having bodily and mental autonomy (Articles 3, 4, 9, 12, 13, 18, 19, 20)
- reason and autonomy are inalienable (Articles 2, 6, 7)
- the denial of another's reason and autonomy is dehumanising (Articles 5, 30)

The latter include:

- law (Articles 6, 8, 10, 11, 14)
- nationality (Article 15)
- family (Article 16)
- economic security (Articles 22, 25)
- intellectual property and land ownership (Articles 17, 27)
- government participation (Article 21)
- community (Articles 27, 28, 29, 30)
- education (Article 26)
- physical health and well-being (Article 25)
- leisure time (Article 24)
- fair work (Article 23)

These conditions of humanity happen-in-place; without a guarantee of place, human rights are a meaningless proposition. This happening-in-place is, again, not a mere co-locatedness of humans in public and private spaces where civic functions and daily life are carried out. Place is the designation of self within a wider world. It is the experience and expression of autonomy, belonging, and identity.[5] It is how we draw a boundary between self and non-self.[6] It does not end with the outlines of our bodies but includes the environment within which that body moves and which the ego utilises for its aims. The space of a place might have measurable extension but, like light, simultaneously occupies a second state in the mind as a part of one's own body. A disoriented human with nowhere to be loses their reason to vertigo and the anxiety of survival.[7] A social humanity is impossible without a guaranteed place in which to be and stay: the radical British geographer Doreen Massey writes, "[S]ociety is necessarily constructed spatially, and that fact – the spatial organization of society – makes a difference to how it works" (Massey, 1992, p. 70). In the declaration's model, however, one's rights, and thus one's personhood, have no spatial existence. Only the prospect of land ownership and abstract right to housing nod to the a priori condition of human existence in time and space.

Phenomenology is the study of first-person experience and considers the quality of an embodied where-ness as integral to a self-concept. While psychoanalysis puts less emphasis on external reality as a point of investigation, it is also a phenomenology of mental contents that considers an ego, or self, as originating from a somatic experience of the world. Freud writes in *The Ego and the Id* that "The ego is first and foremost a bodily ego. . . . [I]t is itself the projection of a surface" (Freud, 1961b, p. 26). Both are in contrast to the Enlightenment-era concepts that tie human selfhood to awareness and consciousness, with body and space as something altogether external to it (Casey, 2001, p. 683). If we apply both methodologies to thinking about an agreement that protects selfhood, it becomes impossible to ignore the need for a literally grounded one. In his essay "Building, Dwelling, Thinking," Heidegger considers how the human be-ing is indistinguishable from *dwelling*, or staying in a place (Heidegger, 1971). One cannot exist bodily or mentally without being aware of the fourfold: earth, sky, mortality, and divinity.[8] As the Australian philosopher Jeff Malpas interprets Heidegger's ideas, "Place is not founded *on* subjectivity but that *on* which subjectivity is founded" (p. 35). Thus, the true nature of building is not simply the erecting of structures to contain our human activity but is in the consideration of ourselves as being somewhere in particular that allows us to exist. Heidegger also notes that in the act of thinking about anything, one is already "there" with it (Heidegger, 1971). This embedded there-ness is what might account for the experience of homesickness: a sudden recognition of the discontinuity in one's places of being in the context of familiar routines. As the child of immigrants from India to the United States, I recall a feeling of slippage between places in my family's everyday life. Our habits could feel determined by the dictates of a different location than the one we were actually in, leading to the feeling of living somehow parallel to and elsewhere from the people around us. This ghostliness of a lost place is apparent, I think, in this vignette I recall from growing up:

> Standing in the kitchen one day, my father remarked, disappointed, that "this is not a cucumber." He was holding a slice of bland watery vegetable, puzzled. It was not in fact *kheera*, the Indian variety of the same species, which is crunchy and bitter. Strangely, it was not the first time he'd had a cucumber from America, though perhaps the one he now held was particularly tasteless. His exclamation spurred a conversation between he and my mother about how America is so different from India. The *kheera* bought from the peddler every morning in Delhi was picked shortly before it was sold. This waxy, fat thing my parents beheld was adamantly not. They were both suddenly overcome by loss, somewhat paralyzed, holding the cucumber that was not a *kheera*.

In this moment between my parents, the cucumber/*kheera* revealed itself not as just the object of a hunger drive, but as containing time, loss, and the entire distance between an Indian street cart and an American supermarket. At that moment, not only were they both disoriented, but had also briefly lost a sense of self. Interestingly, they chose to keep buying cucumbers instead of adapting Indian meals to better-tasting local produce, perhaps as a protest against assimilation.

A psychoanalytic interpretation of the idea of *dwelling* could be that *dwelling* is as much of an instinct as aggression. *Dwelling* could be considered as manifested through a *drive to build* – a self through place-structures as much as through human attachments or eating. In his description of satisfactory parental care, Winnicott refers to the concept of "holding." In this initial stage of a parent-child relationship, he takes holding to mean not only holding of the baby, but the provision of the total environment of the baby, *which is a "three-dimensional or space relationship with time gradually added in"* (Winnicott, 1960, p. 589). This holding phase is associated with the development of the baby into an individual, with a mind, and requires the presence of a reliable, good-enough environment (Winnicott, 1960, p. 590). Winnicott goes on to describe other phases of the parent-child relationship required for the baby's maturation; however, he does not come back to the concept of the "space relationship" in his work. But this requirement never disappears, as the geographers and phenomenologists note – it must, at some point, be taken over by the developing infant. Winnicott takes the capacity to be alone as a central achievement of mental development. A stable inner space is created through the introjected ego-supportive environment initially provided by the parent, allowing the ego to provide for itself (Winnicott, 1958, p. 420). I suggest *dwelling, as a capacity to maintain a relationship with external space,* is the maturational endpoint of the *drive to build.* The ability to *dwell* is necessary for complete human development. A baby comes to be, via its parent, through its psyche, soma, *and* the earth upon which it is born. We are cognitive and embodied and require *a somewhere in which to be both.* This capacity cannot bloom without a place in which one can stay.

The satisfaction of the instinct to dwell through a drive to build is, in my opinion, being *at home.* Not only, as Heidegger discusses, upon the earth, but in in a specific place whose shape and forms are familiar. In *Civilization and Its Discontents,* Freud provides a famous meditation in which he compares the mind and its contents to the eternally excavated city of Rome. The ego at first contains everything and only later separates the external world from itself. But, like Rome's ruins, traces of the ego's original history might still be found, in which an ancient oceanic feeling of merger with the world resides (p. 67–69). If the ego contains all, and eventually differentiates internal and external, then this separation of contents need not be limited: why do we assume the ego comes to contain only thoughts, feelings, or the sensations of our own bodies? Babies make use of the mother's breast and initially do not know it as separate; over time, the infant does come to understand the breast as belonging to its mother. As the breast becomes simultaneously an internal and external object, states of mourning, guilt, love, and hate occur towards it. These relations build the ego (Klein, 1946, p. 105). Likewise, the baby must internalise a relationship with a home so that it will be able to have an embodied ego that can dwell. *Holding* occurs in a *home* – a place that is reliably there, like its parent. *Home* has stable perceived physical characteristics over time, like the breast. The infant would come to know the home as itself, as it does initially with the breast and the entire world.

Thus, human development dwells within a home. That home, like the breast, must be consistently available for the gratification of a dwelling drive. The condition required for this is the possibility of *staying in a place.* Otherwise, the infant risks becoming a person who cannot stay anywhere (and is deprived of an essential aspect of selfhood. Wim Dekkers, in a paper on the phenomenology of home in dementia care, considers that people "have a body and are a body at the same time" and that the body is a "source of selfhood that does not derive its agency from a cognitive form of knowledge" (Dekkers, p. 292). He reflects on how the loss of mind coincides with feeling lost in space because apraxia destroys the *habitual bodily familiarity* (emphasis my own) bred from tasks organised within the physical contours of a home. This parallels the concept of the "skin ego," as elaborated by French psychoanalyst Didier Anzieu. The skin ego is "a representation of the boundary between the internal world and environment" (Anzieu-Premmereur, 2015, p. 659). Through the reception and creation of sensations, the skin provides a unity of contact with the mother and forms an envelope for psychic contents (Anzieu-Premmereur, 2015, p. 660). It follows that the built and natural elements of space organise the body and, with it, our mental states. Routine spatial experience is a container, like skin contact. In this way, selfhood is constituted by the organisation of one's body in space through the physicality of being at home, as it is also eventually through rationality, cognition, or mental contents. Over time, one develops their own capacity for being at home, by becoming able to utilise a place through which to sustain their life – by working, creating, socialising, eating, and participating in communal activity. Being at home can occur over a large geography that encompasses not only where one sleeps at night but one's neighbourhood or even a city.

In *Civilization and Its Discontents*, Freud regards what is forgotten in the mind as not destroyed. He also draws an analogy between trauma to and inflammation of the brain to the demolitions and replacements of buildings (p 71). The physical forms of a place which are destroyed cannot be forgotten. They are missed, grieved lost objects, aspects of ego which can never be accessed again except in dreams and memory. There is pain in such loss, akin to the loss of the breast, perhaps more so – as there is less pressure to separate the space of the home from oneself than to separate from the breast. Indeed, the mother may withdraw her breast, but home is always a communal situation. Losing the structures of home and other aspects of a familiar built environment might even be similar to bodily trauma. Home, mother, breast, family, body, earth, and sky comprise our human-ness.

Staying in place is as much a requirement for human growth and development as are food, water, and other conditions that allow for bodily and psychological integrity. There is a relationship between a person, their human potential, and the natural and built forms of the external world; to deny this, I say, is dehumanising. Centring geographical stability as a prerequisite for healthy mental development also problematises current systems of capital and land ownership. Migration and forced displacement are considered traumatising events - the loss of control over one's immediate geography ought to be as well. A lack of say over land use in one's community, for example, could be considered a deprivation of a person's humanity as could be the forces of unchecked gentrification. In this context, I invite readers to consider the development projects underway not only globally, but in their own towns and cities: Do the cost-benefit analyses conducted by officials include the psychological toll of a transformed streetscape or altered skyline? To whom do the proposed benefits flow from the wreckage that occurs? Will what comes next provide a facilitating environment? Will the spaces that evolve allow for mirroring and self-efficacy, vital functions that allow a person to develop agency and ownership of their lived experience? What is being done in towns and cities to protect the living spaces of people threatened by economic hardship, climate change, and global conflict? Loss is ineluctable, but the traumatic deprivation of autonomy and reason through geopolitical displacement should not be.

Notes

1 I use the word "mother" as opposed to "primary caregiver" to capture associations to the psychological containment functions often described as "maternal" in psychoanalytic literature. The word "mother" is not meant to imply that such caretaking functions are gendered or that a birth/biological parent is the only one who can provide such functions.
2 Eminent domain is the right of a government to expropriate private property for public use with payment of compensation. It was widely used post-WWII throughout major American cities for urban renewal projects that razed slums, often in inner city areas with high concentrations of African American people, to encourage the development of higher-income housing and businesses.
3 Per a March 2021 report from the Council on Foreign Relations, more than one million Uighurs, a mostly Muslim, Turkic-speaking ethnic group in China's Xinjiang province, have been removed from their homes and 65% of the mosques in the region destroyed.
4 According to Land Conflict Watch (Gupta, 2017), the Mandal Dam project in Jharkhand, India, led to the deliberate destruction of 32 tribal villages when the gates of the incomplete dam were opened to drive away protesters whose land had been appropriated. The Ilisu Dam was completed in 2020 in Hasankeyf, an ancient Silk Road town in Turkey. Seventy-thousand people were displaced, and villages and Neolithic-era sites destroyed. A person interviewed for the article sadly noted, "They made migrants of us."
5 Melinda Milligan (Milligan, M 2003) considers how the emotional experience of nostalgia is an attempt to repair identity discontinuity caused by involuntary disruptions of place attachment.
6 As climate change forces people from ancestral homes, a community of Native Americans on the sinking land of Isle-de-Jean-Charles describes the anxieties related to the loss of a way of being with the physical world in the *New York Times* (Davenport, C 2016).
7 The *New York Times* reported the story of a farmer who committed suicide by lighting his house on fire while barricaded inside when authorities came to remove him from his land. The farm had been appropriated for the construction of a highway (Barry E 2021).
8 Adam Bobeck in his translation of *Being dwelling thinking* explains that some have interpreted the fourfold to mean spatiality (earth and sky) and temporality (divinity and mortality). Heidegger, M. (1951).

References

Anzieu-Premmereur, C. (2015). The skin-ego: Triadic sensuality, trauma in infancy and adult narcissistic issues. *The Psychoanalytic Review, 102*(5), 659–681.

Barry, E. (2021, May 27). Goodbye to a yankee farmer, the ghost of exit 8. *NYT*.

Casey, E. (2001). Between geography and philosophy: What does it mean to be in the place-world? *Annals of the Association of American Geographers, 91*(4), 683–693.

Davenport, C., & Robertson, C. (2016, May 2). Resettling the first American 'climate refugees'. *NYT*.

Dekkers, W. (2011). Dwelling, house and home: Towards a home-led perspective on dementia care. *Med Health Care and Philos, 14*, 291–300.

Freud, S. (1961a). Civilization and its discontents. In J. Strachey (Trans.), *The complete psychological works of Sigmund Freud* (Vol. XXI, pp. 64–145). London: Hogarth Press.

Freud, S. (1961b). The ego and the id. In J. Strachey (Trans.), *The complete psychological works of Sigmund Freud* (Vol. XIX, pp. 13–140). London: Hogarth Press.

Fullilove, M. (2005). *Root shock: How tearing up city neighborhoods hurts America and what we can do about it*. New York: One World Books.

Gall, C. (2020, July 5). An ancient valley lost to 'progress'. *NYT*.

Gupta, A. (2017, March 30). Families displaced by Mandal Dam in Jharkhand oppose project resumption. *Land Conflict Watch*. Retrieved from www.landconflictwatch. org/conflicts/mandal-dam-displaced-people-angry-over-re-construction-plan

Heidegger, M. (1951). *Being dwelling thinking* (A. Bobeck, Trans.). Retrieved from www.academia.edu/34279818/Building_Dwelling_Thinking_by_Martin_Heidegger_Translation_and_Commentary_by_Adam_Bobeck_

Heidegger, M. (1971). Being dwelling thinking. In A. Hofstadter (Trans.), *Poetry, language, thought*. New York: Harper Colophon Books.

Klein, M. (1946). Notes on some schizoid mechanisms. *International Journal of Psychoanalysis, 27*(3–4), 99–110.

Koegel, P., Melamid, E., & Burnam, M. A. (1995, December). Childhood risk factors for homelessness among homeless adults. *American Journal of Public Health, 85*(12), 1642–1649.

Maizland, L. (2021, March). China's repression of Uyghurs in Xinjiang. *Council on Foreign Relations*. Retrieved from www.cfr.org/backgrounder/chinas-repression-uyghurs-xinjiang

Malpas, J. (1998). Finding place: Spatiality, locality and subjectivity. In A. Light & J. Smith (Eds.), *Philosophies of place* (pp. 21–43). Lanham, MD: Rowman and Littlefield.

Massey, D. (1992, November–December). Politics and space/time. *NLR, 196*, 66–84.

Milligan, M. J. (2003, Summer). Displacement and identity discontinuity: The role of nostalgia in establishing new identity categories. *Symbolic Interaction, 26*(3), 381–340.

Samnøy, A. (1993, May). *Human rights as international consensus: The making of the universal declaration of human rights 1945–1948*. Bergen, Norway: Michelsen Institute.

Winnicott, D. W. (1958, September–October). The capacity to be alone. *International Journal of Psychoanalysis, 39*(5), 416–420.

Winnicott, D. W. (1960). The theory of the parent-infant relationship. *International Journal of Psychoanalysis, 41*, 585–595.

Index

Note: Page numbers in *italics* indicate a figure on the corresponding page. Page numbers followed by "n" indicate a note.

For Product Safety Concerns and Information please contact our EU
representative GPSR@taylorandfrancis.com
Taylor & Francis Verlag GmbH, Kaufingerstraße 24, 80331 München, Germany

9 7 8 1 0 3 2 0 6 6 5 2 3